Our Bodies Are Selves

Our Bodies Are Selves

Philip Hefner, Ann Milliken Pederson,
and Susan Barreto

CASCADE *Books* • Eugene, Oregon

OUR BODIES ARE SELVES

Copyright © 2015 Philip Hefner, Ann Milliken Pederson, and Susan Barreto. All rights reserved. Except for brief quotations in critical publications or reviews, no part of this book may be reproduced in any manner without prior written permission from the publisher. Write: Permissions, Wipf and Stock Publishers, 199 W. 8th Ave., Suite 3, Eugene, OR 97401.

Cascade Books
An Imprint of Wipf and Stock Publishers
199 W. 8th Ave., Suite 3
Eugene, OR 97401

www.wipfandstock.com

ISBN 13: 978-1-60899-843-2

Cataloguing-in-Publication Data

Hefner, Philip J.

Our bodies are selves / Philip Hefner, Ann Milliken Pederson, and Susan Barreto

X + Y p. ; 23 cm. Includes bibliographical references.

ISBN 13: 978-1-60899-843-2

1. Theological anthropology. 2. Human body (Philosophy). 3. Religion and science. I. Pederson, Ann. II. Barreto, Susan. III. Title.

B105.B64 H44 2015

Manufactured in the U.S.A. 07/30/2015

P. H.—to Neva.

A. M. P.—to Gary.

S. B.—to my parents, Gerald and Violet.

Contents

Acknowledgments | ix
Abbreviations | x

1. **A New Paradigm: Body-Self** | 1
   Philip Hefner and Ann Milliken Pederson

2. **Getting Around: Disability and Life in the Spirit** | 11
   Philip Hefner

3. **Personal Narrative: Living in the Middle Years** | 29
   Ann Milliken Pederson

4. **In the Early Years: Tiny Promises** | 44
   Susan Barreto

5. **Discovering Our Culture's Script:**
   A Manifesto about Our Cultural Views of Bodyselves | 58
   Ann Milliken Pederson

6. **Where Medicine and Christianity Collide** | 76
   Ann Milliken Pederson

7. **A Scientific Take on Our Bodyselves:**
   What Science Tells Us about Our Bodies and Ourselves | 104
   Philip Hefner

8. **The Human Journey** | 122
   Philip Hefner

9. **Nature, Mystery, and God** | 136
   Philip Hefner

**10 Luther on the Body:
  Incarnation, Sacrament, Technoself, and Faith** | 155
   Ann Milliken Pederson

11 The Body of Christ | 162
   Ann Milliken Pederson

Afterword | 189

Suggestions for Further Reading | 191
Bibliography | 195

Acknowledgments

AS WITH ALL OF life, writing this book was a collaborative project. In many ways, the book demands more from us, but our bodyselves have had enough for now. We are exceedingly grateful to the following people and institutions that have helped us along the way and we offer our gratitude:

To Lynn Kauppi whose meticulous editing and keen eye to detail has been invaluable.

To Augustana College and the Augustana Artist and Research Fund for supporting this project.

To Karie Frank, at Augustana College, who did initial preparation and editing on the manuscript.

To the faculty on the Section of Ethics and Humanities at the Sanford School of Medicine at the University of South Dakota, especially to LuAnn Eidsness, Jerome Freeman, Ellie Schellinger, and Mary Helen Harris for all their guidance related to medicine and bioethics.

To the many colleagues and friends who have read and commented on the manuscript: Paul Sponheim, Michelle Bartel, Paul Rohde, Ellen Noth, Kim Beckman, Kristin Largen.

To our families, we are especially grateful.

Abbreviations

GENERAL

bya	billion years ago
DNA	deoxyribonucleic acid
ELCA	Evangelical Lutheran Church in America
ELCC	Evangelical Lutheran Church in Canada
ELW	*Evangelical Lutheran Worship* [Evangelical Lutheran Church in America and Evangelical Lutheran Church in Canada. Minneapolis: Augsburg Fortress, 2006.]
IAAF	International Association of Athletics Federation
IVF	in vitro fertilization
KJV	King James Version
LW	*Luther Works*
MRI	magnetic resonance imaging
mya	million years ago
NICU	neonatal intensive care unit
NRSV	New Revised Standard Version
PET scan	positron emission tomography scan
TH	Transhumanist Movement

SCRIPTURE

1 Cor	1 Corinthians
Col	Colossians
Eccl	Ecclesiastes
Gen	Genesis
Job	Job
Lev	Leviticus

Abbreviations

Luke	Gospel of Luke
Ps	Psalm
Rom	Romans
Song	Song of Songs (also known as Song of Solomon)

1

A New Paradigm
Body-Self

Philip Hefner and Ann Milliken Pederson

> ... to access my body in a more living and engaged way, I needed a paradigm shift. I had to literally change my relationship to the world.
> MATTHEW SANFORD, *WAKING: A MEMOIR OF TRAUMA AND TRANSCENDENCE*

WE ARE EXPLORING A change in how we think and how we relate to our world as we learn to live as embodied persons, engaging our bodies, listening to them, and listening as well to our Christian traditions of faith. We are on a journey: one that begins with the body, traverses several landscapes, and returns to where we started, our bodies now understood in new ways that point to the paradigm shift we seek. We are persuaded that on this journey of accessing our bodies, we are companions along the journey of God's incarnation in the world.

We think of this book as a conversation-starter about the Christian notion of incarnation, or the central tenet to our faith that God took on human flesh in the person of Jesus Christ. It has been a fruitful starting point for us the authors, and we hope for you the reader as well. There's a conversation here to be had with oneself, and every theme we touch upon may well trigger an interior back-and-forth, leading even to a wider conversation.

Our focus is on body: my body, your body. This should be simple and straight-forward; after all, *body* is very *in* right now, trendy, even. Everywhere we look—TV, movies, magazines, the internet, in all forms of advertising—bodies are at the center. But this centrality of body does not make it simple to understand. In fact, the centrality of the body betrays how fragmented our self-understanding really is. Our very language points to this fragmentation.

At the heart of our quest for the paradigm there nestles an idea that beckons, a kind of Holy Grail if you will, that we attempt to understand and sketch. We call this the idea of *bodyself*. In its essence, bodyself asserts that my body is my very self and that myself is a body. Our dictionary, as well as our encyclopedia of ideas, rests on the assumption that body and self are two separate things. After all, the words and ideas that we work with are expressions of our culture, a culture that is deeply informed by a worldview of body/self separation. The reasons for this separation are not difficult to understand: I look at my body and see that it is finite, it is bounded, and it grows weary, is subject to disease, deteriorates, and dies. But that is not my essential self, because I can in my imagination go places my body has never been; I can dream of worlds that have never existed.

Matthew Sanford, an inspirational speaker, author, and yoga instructor, who was paralyzed from the waist down following an automobile accident, marks the goal for us: "*to access my body in a more living and engaged way, I needed a paradigm shift. I had to literally change my relationship to the world.*"[1] That's what we're after, a new paradigm. As we seek out this new paradigm, we find it is an elusive thing, and that will be evident as we move through the successive chapters of this book. It is not just that the paradigm is hard to grasp, it's also that our language isn't up to the task we face—nor are our ideas. Our dictionary does not contain the words we need, and our encyclopedia of concepts lacks adequate resources for our thinking. For example, when a friend suffers from clinical depression, we say that they have a mental illness. We are discovering that our mind, or that which is mental, is not simply confined to the brain, or separate from our bodies, yet we struggle with naming what we call mental illness. If someone is diagnosed

---

1. Sandford, *Waking*, 149.

with diabetes, we don't tell others that they have a physical illness, and yet diabetes affects the whole person. While what we hope for as authors is a paradigm that challenges the dualisms we have inherited about body and self, mental and physical, self and other, we know that we are caught in the trap of our own cultural expressions which are not adequate to the sense of who we really are as created in the image of God. And to further complicate our task, the sciences and social media (as just two examples) move so rapidly through the shifting boundaries of self and other, self and body that we hardly have time to reflect on the changes.

For hundreds of years, we have talked about body, mind, spirit, and soul—names for ideas that we construct in order to explain our experience. They have worked for us in explaining some of the things we mentioned above—for example, that my body is earthbound, whereas my self can soar to situations and worlds that do not even exist in my present experience. Body, mind, and soul are products of reflection trying to make sense of the experience that is me. This duality of body and mind has a venerable history; today it is institutionalized in our philosophy and science—relating body and soul, brain and mind, has become an industry in itself, analyzed in thousands of learned books and articles.

A basic separation, a deep-down devaluing of body is embedded in our cultural experience, and it shapes how we as individuals view our own bodies. This devaluing is expressed in a bodyself separation that has conditioned us profoundly—from which, we are convinced, by our own experience and by conversations with many other people, it is extraordinarily difficult to free ourselves. Over the ages, our common conversation has separated *body* and *self* so thoroughly that it is very difficult to bring the two together in a meaningful way. At the outset, we must acknowledge that this separation is quite understandable. It grows out of experience that is real and also widespread—even universal. This experience and the motives for interpreting it in terms of bodyself separation are not always negatives, nor do they always cause harm. We want to make this clear as we approach the themes of this book. We want to make two points, however: (1) that the idea of separation is at odds with our wider scientific and religious understandings, and (2) if carried forward in certain exaggerated ways, separation thinking can close off important experience and insights, and it can be very destructive. As we reflect on this separation-thinking, we recognize that it is inextricably part of our own thinking—we do not write as if we are immaculately liberated from it. Thinking in terms of a separation between body and self challenges us to provide better interpretations of our experience as bodies who are also selves, or selves who are embodied—*bodyselves*.

There are two fundamental motifs that underlie this perspective of separation. The first is the *motif of the essential self*. The term "essential self" is "the kind of thing human beings have had in mind, over thousands of years, in talking of 'my inmost self'; 'my self, my inward self'; the 'living, central, inmost I'; the 'secret self enclosed within.'"[2] Throughout the centuries, different body parts have been identified as this essential self: the chamber of the heart, the gut, the breath of life, and now the brain with each part metaphor and literal, locating who we are within our body as the essential core of who we are.

This sense of our essential self is vividly expressed in news accounts of Brendan Marrocco, the first veteran of the wars in Iraq and Afghanistan to lose all four limbs in combat and survive. The twenty-six-year-old infantryman lost all four limbs in a 2009 roadside bomb attack in Iraq, The language of a 2010 *New York Times* article speaks volumes about the struggle to relate body and self. The headline of the article gives a hint of the issues: "Spirit Intact, Soldier Reclaims His Life."[3] Despite horrible damage to his body, his "spirit" is intact. The author of the article writes that when his mother got her first look at her son, she "struggled to see beyond the wounds, the respirator and the missing arms and legs." Why should she "see beyond" her son's body? Because in that beyond, his true self could reassure her. The soldier has also met, fallen in love with, and proposed marriage to a young woman who is a member of a volunteer group that visits wounded veterans in the hospital. She is described as a person who sees "what is there rather than what is missing"—a very suggestive use of words, because they imply that the disabled man she saw led her to see more deeply just who he is. Can we say that she did not have to look beyond his body, because she saw more deeply into his body? Perhaps it is the author's struggle that is more accurately expressed here, since she goes on to write that the fiancé "has a gift: She can see clearly and comfortably past the disfigurement and disabilities." Apparently the injured man's self is visible only to those who have a gift for seeing past or beyond the body. The condition of the body may be considered an obstacle for the self. In her own words, the fiancé's comments are more richly suggestive as she responds to the family's concern that her actions are motivated by pity and that "empathy was overriding

2. Strawson, *Selves*, 8.
3. Alvarez, "Spirit Intact."

common sense": "'Do you really love him? Do you pity him?' There is no reason to pity him. He had a horrible thing happen to him. But he is no less of a person." We focus on the language that is used in this article, because whether it is more reflective of the author's state of mind or that of the soldier's mother and fiancé, it expresses poignantly the dilemma we all face when we think about the relationship of body to self. The soldier who has lost all four of his limbs poses an unusual, we might say, extreme case, but precisely in such a case we recognize the issues we all face. The language is imprecise; it does not go as far as we would like in our effort to clarify our dilemma—just as most often language fails us. There is also a subtext of faith in the story, elaborated in terms of the strength of the human spirit in face of the body's devastation. Even miraculous elements are present in the descriptions of the soldier's perseverance, the medical successes, and the love between him and his fiancé.

The comments that readers have made on this article are equally revealing. One commenter, who identifies himself as holding a PhD and being a minister, writes: "He is severely injured, his body shattered, he IS less of a person, and no amount of scientifically enhanced wooden legs will change that."[4] This comment elicited sharp rejoinders, including: "This soldier, with all his limbs missing is more of a man than you will ever be."[5] Also: "You may have Ph.D. credentials but they seem to have betrayed you. This young man seems short on credentials, but his humanism honors his struggle and hopefully will come to his rescue."[6] The forcefulness of all these comments shows in the first case how difficult it is to relate self to body, and in the rejoinders to how passionately the writers want to preserve the soldier's self from the destruction that has befallen his body.

This four-time amputee, we discover, is pursuing his physical therapy with a vigor that impresses his doctors and his therapists. Focusing on his incredible efforts and successes with sophisticated orthotic legs, it seems clear that he is not accepting the idea of separating his self from his body. Whatever hopes and plans he has for his body, he apparently wants his body to participate fully. Mobility of body and our dreams for ourselves go hand-in-hand. They are not separated, they are one. That this oneness is so deeply ingrained in our self-image is testimony to the falsity of ideas that separate body and self.

4. Ibid., comment 8, E. M. Camarena.
5. Ibid., comment 11, J.H.
6. Ibid., comment 62, Ron.

Our Bodies Are Selves

We shall pick up this challenge of how our essential selves relate to our bodies—recognizing how difficult an issue it is.

A second motif speaks of *the body as instrumental,* as a means for achieving other values that are important to us. This view puts great emphasis on our bodies and on the value we place on our body in relationship to others. Fictional stories like *My Sister's Keeper* by Jodi Picoult or *Never Let Me Go* by Kazuo Ishiguro reflect our fear of who we become when we simply treat others as means to our ends—as replacement parts.[7] In *My Sister's Keeper,* Anna, the younger sister who sues her parents for medical emancipation, explains how she came into the world: "They sat me down and told me all the usual stuff, of course—but they also explained that they chose little embryonic me, specifically, because I could save my sister, Kate. 'We loved you even more,' my mother made sure to say, 'because we knew what exactly we were getting.'"[8] The novel became an instant success because, like Anna, most people can understand what it is like to be used for someone else's purposes instead of feeling valued simply for who they are. In this story, body is central to the parents' actions.

Since the condition of our body is a high priority, we treat it as any other valuable object—our cars for example. We keep it buffed, take pains to keep it in good condition, see that it gets regular service and repairs, and we agonize when it doesn't live up to our expectations. Like the things we acquire in our consumption-oriented society, we expect our body to make a statement about who we are—a statement that others will admire and even envy. When our body does not make the statement we wish for, we may become angry, depressed, or even self-debasing—think of anorexia, cutting or obsessive cosmetic surgery, for example. Americans spent almost $12 billion in 2008 for more than 10 million cosmetic procedures—surgical and non-surgical. Even though this strategy takes our body seriously, it makes the body, on the one hand, into a thing apart from the calculating self that manipulates it, and, on the other hand, depicts the body as totally subservient to the wishes of the autonomous self.

The same can be said about the Transhumanist (TH) Movement whose mentality permeates our culture today. In its efforts to extend the human life span, TH approaches our bodies much as if they were automobiles that can be rebuilt to extend their mileage. In the TH perspective, however, the body serves a desire to extend the length of life. Further, many in the TH

---

7. Picoult, *My Sister's Keeper*; Ishiguro, *Never Let Me Go*.
8. Picoult, *My Sister's Keeper*, 8.

movement are artificial intelligence researchers, who seem to show an almost gnostic contempt for the human body. "You're stuck in the mire of pig shit. All of us are. You've got to be free of that. You've got to become pure mind," stated programmer and hacker Charles Lect.[9] The robotics and artificial intelligence researcher Hans Moravec sees a human being "as the *pattern* and the *process* going on in my head and body, not the machinery supporting that process. If the process is preserved, I am preserved. The rest is mere jelly."[10] Such researchers desire nothing more than to upload the contents of human minds from its container—the brain, encased in the body—into robots capable of artificial intelligence, thus releasing the mind from imprisoning human flesh. This objectifying emphasis on the body as a thing to be manipulated is not what we intend in our focus on body. In this book, our view of the body is not instrumental, as if the body exists solely to promote other ends and values.

In the so-called "wellness movement," which is fostered by many businesses and other organizations, caring for the body serves as a means to reducing medical expenses and therefore the financial outlay for health insurance. Even church bodies who consider it progressive to recognize the place of the body have fallen into this instrumental mode of thinking. In researching the background of three large Protestant denominations' emphasis on wellness, we discovered that the program originated in the denomination's agency that deals with health insurance. With the best of intentions, that agency proposed to the denominational governing board that an emphasis on wellness might stem the ominously increasing demands on the health insurance offered by the denomination. Churches often underscore that clergy perform their duties better if they maintain healthy behaviors. This instrumental approach is not necessarily wrong or evil, but it is at bottom a demeaning of the body as such. It is certainly not adequate for comprehending the depth dimension of our existence as bodies who are selves.

My body can be disabled, paralyzed, lose body parts through amputation, but myself goes on—imagining, creating, relating to other people, compensating for my body's limitations as I carry on my life. My body lives its life close to the ground, while my self is a high-flier, not limited to a nose-to-the-ground existence.

9. Fjermedal, *The Tomorrow Makers*, 199.
10. Moravec, *Mind Children*, 117.

This self of mine is very precious. It has integrity, is aware of moral obligations, engages in acts of love and caring, and recognizes other selves, as well. To go even further, my self relates to a higher power, to God. My self is reckoned as precious to those other selves, and even more profoundly, to God. It seems appropriate to speak of the precious center of my self as my *spirit* and also as my *soul*. It seems obvious that my self's core identity, as well as its significance and meaningfulness are not coterminous with my body; a deep chasm separates them.

Nevertheless, in light of our experience, our scientific knowledge, and our Christian faith, we believe that this worldview of separation, understandable though it be, is inadequate. Our dictionary and our encyclopedia of ideas were compiled so as to make this dominant worldview understandable, to provide the basic ideas and the words to express them. Little wonder that a shift in understanding, an attempt to frame a new paradigm, will have to compile its own new encyclopedia and construct a dictionary to go with it.

As we proceed, we come to see even the idea of *body* is strange. In my most fundamental awareness, I simply *am*; I feel, see, smell, hear, taste; I also think, make judgments, know pleasure and pain, joy and fear, attraction and repulsion. I definitely do not have a sense that I am a spirit or a mind encased in a body. When I look at my hand, I see myself, not a body. When I cut my finger, it is not something called my body that hurts, it is me, myself. In that moment of pain there is no separation, no mind or soul mired in human flesh, just the oneness of me, myself.

The new paradigm we seek is no less reflective than the body-soul paradigm, but it retains a fundamental oneness. We're helped by an aphorism heard years ago from a friend: "Mind is what the brain does." We want to rephrase it as, "Myself is what my body does." This aphorism accomplishes two things: it roots myself in my body, and it revises traditional views of body-mind with an explosiveness and an expansiveness that can take us into the new paradigm of *bodyself*.

Bodyself is both a given and a work-in-progress that has yet to be attained. It is a given in that it is our first, primal awareness of ourselves; it is a work-in-progress in that it is not easy to grasp, even harder to talk about. We are so conditioned by our heritage of body and mind as two separate things that it is difficult for us to let a new set of ideas shape our self-understanding. We use external ideas and words to guide and shape our subordinated bodies, rather than listening to the struggle of our bodyselves to form the ideas. We tend to think that our bodies are *object* and as such we need to apply our best knowledge and our religious truth to them. But our bodies are also *subject;* they are seeking knowledge and truth. We are not using our bodies and brains to seek understanding, just as we are not using our bodies to write this book. It is our bodies that are seeking and perceiving truth; it is our bodies that are writing.

The idea of bodyself is also both vision and challenge—vision because it is not yet fully real to us, not in our linguistic expression, not in our conceptualizations, and not in our personal awareness of ourselves; challenge, because as we will discover as our book unfolds, our scientific knowledge, our classic theology, and our experience require the new paradigm of bodyself. In our journey toward the new paradigm, we will at times see through a glass darkly, we will contradict the very bodyself oneness that we aim for—after all, our dictionary is still composed mostly of the words from bygone eras.

We have said that we are initiating a conversation about our bodyselves. How do we converse about ourselves? Where do we start? If you have attempted to write a personal memoir or autobiography, you recognize that it's a tricky business—on several counts.

For one thing, there are many perspectives to consider. We have a professional life, a career—most resumes and obituaries focus on this aspect. But I am also a social being, with a family and friends who have a perspective on me that my professional colleagues may rarely see. I have a psychological life—ups and downs, highs and lows—that is right at the center of myself, kept very private, perhaps only known to my counselors and most intimate friends. What about my personal history—childhood, in which the foundations of self are laid, adolescence, and the rest of my biography?

Besides these various lives (professional, social, psychological), there is the storyline of our life as a whole. Where does the story begin and where does one bring the story to a stop? Everything is refracted through the lens of today, where I stand at this moment, and the story is by no means linear in its unfolding. We do not experience our lives as a movement from A to Z, as if we were starting at Go on the game board and proceeding by steps, space by space, to the end. Many great novelists and poets—James Joyce in *Ulysses,* for example—have abandoned this A to Z format, but a non-fiction book can follow no other format. While our lives only rarely experience the heights and depths of great literature, our lives do follow a course of

S-curves and switchbacks, and the telescoping of past, present, and future just as surely as the scripted lives of fictional characters.

Multiple perspectives and nonlinear storyline merge in our reflections on our bodyselves and in our attempts to understand them. We warn you now not to be misled by the one-chapter-after-another format of this book. The reader would do well, as the book unfolds, to consider each chapter as a fragment of a film script. When you have finished reading, take some time to construct the storyline as seems most meaningful to you, filling in with the scripts you supply from your own story. Finally, keep in mind that the story is about you as bodyself, not a self separated from body, not a self inside a body, but a *bodyself*. While we hope to explore new paradigms for interpreting the landscape of our bodyselves, we realize that our journey seems as much like science fiction as what the journalist reports from the front lines. What the "hot button" topics in the media reflect are the images from our past, images of who we are and where we are going in the future. Part of the problem and possibility of what we are trying to do is that we are characters in our own crazy storyline and we embody multiple perspectives as authors and we also know that we cannot speak for all the characters whose lives are linked to ours.

2

Getting Around
Disability and Life in the Spirit

Philip Hefner

For me, it's all about mobility.[1] Since, until very recently, I was so favored as to be virtually without pain, it's the challenge of getting around. "Disabled" or "handicapped" are abstractions that take shape for me in what politically correct jargon might call "mobility-challenged." This is my personal story, not a treatise on disability; I try to avoid generalizations. Not that generalizations shouldn't be made, but since it is individuals who are struck with infirmity and each one has a distinctive story, abstractions must always be held accountable according to their impact on actual persons. If my story has broader relevance, so much the better, but it begins in the particularities of my own life. That having been said, I believe that living disabled is in some ways an epitome of being human—a pattern that we all will follow at some point in our lives, whether defined as disabled or not. More about this later. I say this as one who has lived most of his life without disability; disability clamped itself on me only within the past seven years.

Psalm 139 has been a favorite passage of Scripture for me. Over the years, I have read it for its inspirational insights, particularly its description

---

1. Throughout this essay, I equate "disability" and "handicapped" with mobility impairment.

of how tightly God holds us: "You hem me in, behind and before, and lay your hand upon me" (v. 5).

> O Lord, you have searched me and known me.
> You know when I sit down and when I rise up;
> > you discern my thoughts from far away.
> You search out my path and my lying down,
> > and are acquainted with all my ways. . . .
> For it was you who formed my inward parts;
> > you knit me together in my mother's womb.
> I praise you, for I am fearfully and wonderfully made.
> Wonderful are your works;
> > that I know very well.
> My frame was not hidden from you,
> when I was being made in secret,
> > intricately woven in the depths of the earth.
> Your eyes beheld my unformed substance.
> In your book were written all the days that were formed for me,
> > when none of them as yet existed.
>
> (Ps 139:1–3, 13–16)

It is one thing to read this as inspirational poetry; I choose actually to believe it and relate it to myself—and that is quite another thing. "You knit me together in my mother's womb"—these are the words that strike me most vividly. In large measure, my story is the story of my body and how it has been knit together.

The Knitter
(June 16, 2012)

"You created every part of me,
knitting me in my mother's womb"—Psalm 139

Knit one purl two
or is it
knit two purl one
can the knitting master
forget
get it wrong
drop a stitch

the warp and the weft
which is which
the weaver's memory
lapses for a moment

a gene here
a gene there
a nucleotide dropped*
or added in
after all, there are
three billion
inside me

the sweater with a
dropped stitch
still goes on sale
as imperfect
irregular
and warms the boy
who never knows
what's dropped
never guesses
the knitter's flawed touch

so the body
with how many
one-billionths
gone askew
has yet outlived
the legendary
three score and ten
mostly unaware
of the knitter's lapse
or is it flawed
can the lost stitch
by design
have been mislaid
the genes with intent

been re-spelled
departing from
the norm
the sweater that
warms with mis-spaced
weave is a different
wrap—not flawed
so the re- or dis-
ordered As and Cs
and Gs and Ts**
make a different
body, not junk
and that body's
reach is its own
sure grasp—not
an error

what did the knitter
have in mind

praise the one
who knits

*A nucleotide is a structural unit of DNA and RNA.
**Nucleotides associated with DNA are commonly referred to as A, C, G, and T. A=adenine; C=cytosine; G=guanine; T=thymine. These are called the alphabet of the genetic code.

From the beginning: I was born with spina bifida, and my disability, now at age eighty-two, goes back that far. Focusing on my birth is to lose most of the story, however. Our lives are a process, a narrative that is dynamic and whose surprises defy understanding. For me, the process has been a life-long unfolding revelation of how my body is knit together.

Since I grew up in the polio epidemic of the 1930s and 40s, the neurological damage in my legs was surmised to be due to a mild case of polio. A diagnosis was not urgent, because I was physically active: sandlot games in football, baseball, and basketball, and a high school letter in tennis. A drop-foot really was not that much of a handicap, even though my middle school peers made great sport mimicking it. But then in the early 1970s, our fourth child died at birth of anencephaly, and later in that decade, another daughter, pre-med at the time, wondered if my problem was spina bifida, since anencephaly is the same neural tube defect, occurring at the opposite end of the spinal column. Without examining me further, my doctors thought that made sense. Magnetic resonance imaging (MRI), the basic tool for diagnosing spina bifida, was not available to me; the first MRI body scan of a human being was performed only in 1977, with widespread use coming several years after.

Shortly before I turned sixty-eight, in the summer of 2000, what happened at birth received a name. Suffering severe back pains, I underwent a thorough examination, this time with MRI. The pains turned out to be only a bad sprain from lifting heavy furniture during a move, but the tests disclosed spina bifida with tethered spinal cord. I was not clear what that meant, and since I exhibited no problems, the specialist recommended that nothing be done. That settled it for me, and I pursued the matter no further; my pains went away and I continued as before. I had a spinal defect, with no significant consequences. Five years later that all began to change. My mobility decreased at an alarming rate. I entered the world of high-tech scientific medicine, where a surgeon explained to me that in my mother's womb—when God was knitting me—when I could be described as yet in the "fish stage," my spinal cord remained abnormally anchored or tethered to the base of my spine so that it could not expand. For seventy years, although my active life was not impaired, I carried with me substantial neurological and other physical defects. Serious surgery was called for, not in hopes of correcting the damage, but rather to prevent or slow down further deterioration. The surgery, now performed on infants and young children, or even in utero, was done by a pediatric surgeon. As I lay stretched out in the shape of a "V," face down, the surgical team worked on me for six hours. The lead surgeon tells me that I am the oldest person he knows to have had this procedure.

For five years afterwards, thanks to intensive physical therapy and fitness training, I maintained a level of physical fitness that exceeded my pre-surgery condition. I walked a mile several times each week with no assistance whatsoever. Those were good years; I had a sense of achievement, overcoming the doleful possibilities of serious birth defects, walking free. Those years came to an end as my legs gradually became recalcitrant: they simply wouldn't work very well, despite regular exercise and fitness training, in which I always pushed myself to my limits. I learned, beginning in 2011, what it means to be mobility handicapped. With a walker, I got around, if slowly, on flat surfaces of a few blocks or less with no obstacles. Doors, stairs, ramps, and museums were another story: they required a cane, a wheelchair, and helpful companions. Poor balance and fear of falling made a cane risky for me. In the winter of 2013, things took another turn, when hip pain put me in a wheelchair and set in motion more than eight months of medical investigation. I thought a simple hip replacement was in my future. In fact, the hip problem has proven to be complex, defying diagnosis; after eight tests and multiple rounds of imaging and the consultation of seven doctors. One conclusion came forth: the doctors judged that I was not a candidate for surgery.

Finally, getting a second opinion—more doctors and more tests—with the same conclusion, that my condition was too complex, surgery might only make it worse. Two sets of doctors from two of our finest medical centers agreed on one thing: no surgery for me, and that means no lessening of the pain through hip replacement.

This taught me, in very concrete terms, a number of things that I had more than once written about in abstract terms. Our bodies are not static; they change over time and sometimes very quickly. What has happened to my body is happening to everybody, to one degree or another. The rapid rate of change is not so common. Our image of *self* must be dynamic, ever-changing. This becomes very clear when we recognize that we are bodyselves, since including body into our self-image makes it much more difficult to freeze our *self* into some timeless, unchanging abstraction. Such a freeze is always self-delusion; we should offer thanks to our bodies for saving us from such delusion. In my case, only eight months elapsed between a scan that showed osteoarthritis of the hip and a second scan revealing unexplained pelvic fractures. There's nothing static about those bones, and the doctors are following the clues in much the same way as Sherlock Holmes followed his leads. And they are successful in ruling certain things out—not so able to find out basic causes and remediate those causes.

A blog piece that I wrote in January 2014, shortly after the second scan, expressing my situation, is incorporated in the following paragraphs.

When the Angel Kneads Harshly

What we choose to engage is so tiny!
What engages us is so great!
If only we would let ourselves be dominated

as things do by some immense storm,
we would become strong too, and not need names.
When we win it's with small things,
and the triumph itself makes us small.
What is extraordinary and eternal
does not want to be bent by us.
I mean the Angel who appeared
to the wrestlers of the Old Testament:
when the wrestler's sinews
grew like long metal strings,
he felt them under his fingers
like chords of deep music.
Whoever was beaten by this Angel
(who often simply declined the fight)
went away proudM and strengthened
and great from that harsh hand,
that kneaded him as if to change his shape.
Winning does not tempt that man.
This is how he grows: by being defeated, decisively,
by constantly greater beings.

(Rainer Maria Rilke, "The Man Beholding," translated by Robert Bly, revised by Philip Hefner.)[2]

This poem by Rilke speaks to me particularly, because at the present moment I am wrestling with health issues that are complex and make diagnosis difficult. When the diagnosis is arrived at, the treatment will very likely be comparably complex. The diagnostic processes will contribute new knowledge to my understanding of myself. My experience reinforces the sense I have had for some years that we are always being revealed anew to ourselves, in both our bodies and our spirits.

Rilke's point broke in as revelation to me. In the flash of a moment, I realize that I am caught up in a Jacob-like engagement, not so much with ailments and medical problems as with forces that are larger and more foundational than birth defects, the degeneration that comes naturally to a body that has functioned at the top of its energies for four score years. Hands-on, I am encountering my created nature, my body as the processes

---

2. Hefner, "When the Angel Kneads Harshly."

of nature have shaped it and passed it on to me. My engagement is with more than the sum of my body's medicalized ailments. I am wrestling with my body as it was planted in the soil of evolutionary processes and shaped and circumscribed, kneaded, by those processes. Nature—such an abstract term!—has become concrete and specific in my-body-in-context, which is me. Stream-of-consciousness as a writing style is perhaps the most fitting way to talk about the specificity of nature that makes me what I am at this moment in time.

I say this because my initial condition was spina bifida; and my life in one sense is the story of how my body refused to succumb to the forces that selected against it and, through an amazing set of compensatory processes, carved its shape, sculpted me. Nature allowed and even supported that compensation while exacting the distinctive costs that were entailed. One leg can do the work of two, but not forever. And there is more.

Specific medical issues may be the tiny antagonists that we choose to engage. My present wrestling is with the more fundamental realities of my bodily journey—much of the time, I have not even been aware that they were engaging/kneading me, but I am more aware of their presence now.

Winning is not the issue in this match, growth comes in the defeat. Hard words for us. Fulfillment comes in being the object of the kneading process, not in some imagined triumph over the One who kneads. What could it possibly mean to triumph over the "me-as-incarnated-in-the-chunk-of-nature?" I do not yet understand how strengthening and greatness are bestowed by the harsh hand of the Angel—but I know that understanding will come one day. My identity is being formed. Who I am now throws light on who I have always been, even though I have been unaware of that identity until now.

Words take on new meanings in these days: winning and losing are not what they were. I am seeing new depths in the words of the nineteenth-century theologian's insight that we meet God when we experience utter dependency.[3] I draw closer to that *utter* dependency when I grapple with Rilke's Angel and when I feel that Angel's kneading. Conceding-while-struggling is to become clear about who I am. Is that a loss or a win? Struggling grows out of the insistence that "human" nature has a hand in carving out existence—it is not the Angel alone who wields the sculpting tool. This may be co-creating, an idea I have thought and written about for many years. My self-creation continues, in a way that includes acknowledging

---

3. Schleiermacher, *The Christian Faith*.

the Angel, conceding to the Angel, while never ceasing the struggle. But it is not a struggle against the Angel; it is a struggle for the Angel to acknowledge something as well: no matter how overwhelmed I am, no matter how immeasurably greater the contesting forces are, this dough, this chunk of nature, will take its own shape, even in the face of the ungraspable kneading powers that form my natural and spiritual world. In one sense, my struggle is between me and an Angel Antagonist, while in another, it is a struggle carried on by two allies, two companions—the Angel and I—both of us intent on sculpting a thing of beauty.

Saint Benedict is a resource here: he interpreted Jacob's wrestling ground as holy.[4] *Jacob himself*, as he was kneaded and as he shaped himself, was the point where heaven and earth met, "Jacob's ladder" (Gen 28:10–21). Jacob-sculpted-in-the-grappling-with-the-Angel is the connection.

Grappling, wrestling are rendered in Rilke's German as *Ringen*. (Roll the "R-R-R"!) The physicality of it all is so real—and so fundamentally spiritual. I do not wrestle alone, it is the Angel, along with nature as it expresses itself in me—in all that I have been and shall become—the me that wrestles and is kneaded in the process.[5]

These are the bare physical facts of my story. Not the fullness of who I am by any means, but the bottom line, the ground zero, if you will, of my present life. That bottom line is my body; body is the place I have to start, beginning with each morning's personal rituals, and continuing through mealtime, work, and recreation—keeping in mind during the years of decline that asking someone for help, though frequently necessary, must be a last resort, not a first option. Now, confined to a wheelchair, I am dependent on a night-and-day caregiver. Such dependency has become a spiritual and psychological challenge of its own. All of us live in community, in mutual dependency and self-giving. We take this for granted most of the time.

Handicapped persons never forget their dependency; for them the struggle is discover how they can reciprocate. Body is the object of care and discipline; if the body goes wrong, everyday living must pay the consequences. Body is the weight of flesh to be moved around and bent to many movements and purposes. Moving body through space and time—that's where mobility takes center stage and where disability is the obstacle. How often as I rouse myself from bed or chair, T. S. Eliot's poetic image flashes

---

4. St. Benedict, *The Rule of St. Benedict*, 7:5–9.
5. Hefner, "When the Angel Kneads Harshly."

in my mind: "The broad-backed hippopotamus / Rests on his belly in the mud."[6]

This is all very mundane—even boring. Disability is mundane: ordinary parts of the body that don't work well or don't work at all. Therapy and fitness training focus on these body parts—on the armature that holds the body together and enables it to move. Armature is not exciting, but it looms large in the days of the disabled. Armature is not the life we want to lead; it is the infrastructure that makes that life possible. Having to compensate in dozens of ways for defects in the armature which is so mundane—which should facilitate life, not consume it—this is the source of frustration, and it is tempting to think of it as the enemy of the spirit. Poet Denise Levertov speaks of that which causes the soul to "dwindle sometimes to an ant" scurrying across cracked places where despair lurks, "seething hot and black."[7]

Not always despair, but at the very least frustration. It is precisely this daily tedium of disability that is the challenge. Strangely, when the monotonous rituals of coping take hold so as to become routine, matter-of-fact, and to some extent unconscious—it is in these rare moments that the body becomes free and actually feels a zest for living. This is the moment when awareness of armature fades for a time and it actually serves its purpose. At the same time, body and armature are the clay, not enemy of spirit, but rather that which spirit sculpts. I am always a bodyself.

It may sound as if disability brought me to an obsession with myself, living in my own personal world. In some ways that is the case, but disability also introduced me to a new world outside myself, a world I never dreamed existed. It is a world of high-tech medicine and therapy, populated by fabulously well-trained professionals. It is also a world where people of great thoughtfulness and kindness cross my path every day, some of them known to me, some complete strangers—interspersed with others who seem insensitive and so self-absorbed.

For the movement-impaired disabled, moving toward this freedom is what medical treatment and therapy aim at. Progress does not come without huge technological assists, accompanied by mentors and healers. Surgery, physical therapy and fitness training are labor intensive—and hence expensive. Fitness centers and therapy/exercise equipment are marvels of design and technology. Orthotics (supporting and bracing weak or ineffective joints or muscles), prosthetics (employing artificial devices to replace

---

6. Eliot, "The Hippopotomus," lines 1–2.
7. Levertov, "An Interim," lines 2 and 6, p. 129.

missing parts of the body), canes, crutches, walkers, rollators, wheelchairs, motorized chairs, medi-vans, and kneeling buses are the most publicly visible links in that chain of technology and care giving. Every time disabled men and women walk down the hall or through the streets or into work place or movie theater or concert hall or athletic stadium or church, they are carrying the miracle of that technological assist and personal caring with them in their bones—without it they would not be on the street at all. Though it may not be visible to the average observer, a disabled person is a cyborg, a blending of the organic with the machine—if the technology is not to be seen, it may be hidden inside the body; you can be sure it has played a major role in enabling the disabled to go out in public—indeed it has been essential for survival. It is also true to say that it takes a village to get the disabled moving—a village of healers, therapists, trainers, mentors, friends and family, and the engineers—orthotists and prosthetists who have designed and perfected all kinds of equipment, without which the "hippopotamus" could not get around. We must add the role of the society that is willing to pay the taxes and give the private donations that support the research, training, and applications that the technology and the mentoring require.

The images of cyborg and village bring to mind a number of things. They remind me that as a disabled person, I live within a network that is very personal and intimate while at the same time it is vast and multidimensional with aspects that are by nature impersonal. I am a dependent person in ways that I was unaware of most of my life. This means that I am entwined in relationships—relationships that I must be willing and daring enough to call upon every day if I am to live my life. It is not enough just to be a grateful recipient of the networks.

As expensive as this network of technology and care giving is and as strenuous and time-consuming as it may be to gain the strength and skill to function in this network, it is only the enabler, the prelude to living. To be sure, it is an integral part of living for the disabled, because it may consume hours each day, and while in some respects it has intrinsic value—it is an end in itself—more importantly, it is prerequisite for another goal: to sustain the spirit that makes living possible at a level beyond the nitty-gritty of eating, sleeping, and the rituals of personal hygiene. Living in the everyday world with creativity and élan—the world of creativity, the world of church, with its prayer, praise, and thanksgiving, as well as the world of the theater, the stadium, the mall, and the workplace.

Our Bodies Are Selves

What room does this leave for the spirit, whose presence is the key for life that is more than drudgery? My body has called the tune all along this way—that should be clear. One of the most revelatory, by that I mean mind-opening, dimensions of disability is the way it puts my body inescapably in the forefront of my experience. But my body also has soul—"the active inner part of me that is not shaped by contingencies, that stands free."[8] My soul keeps my spirit alive, and its bottom line is the desire for immortality. Spirit is a constant presence along the way; my body is never separate from my spirit. Here is where things get interesting. I am beginning to understand in my own being something that I have known for some years now in a more detached and theoretical way from the sciences that study the human brain and mind: that my body engages in spiriting. Spirit and body are not two separate entities; my spirit does not enter my body from the outside, nor does it overwhelm my body as a superior power. It's all verbs, not nouns bouncing from one place to another. Rather, my body engages in activity that we call soul or spirituality, even though it really defies capturing in concepts and words. This ensouled flesh (we could also say enfleshed soul) of mine, struggling to bend and move, reflects, relentlessly and deeply, upon itself. It never lets up on itself. It's a thinking body and a spiriting body. My body-spirit urges me to move, to get around. This same body-spirit tells me that my body is not an end in itself—it exists for something! The voice of immortality sounding within me. When I do not or cannot get around, my spirit is sore distressed—I am distressed. And when my final earthly days come, when getting around is no longer the point, because immortality is entering a new phase, I believe that then my spirit will tell me, "It is finished." I believe in the resurrection of the body. The rest is shrouded in mystery.

Relentless spiriting delves deeply as the body probes its condition and its possibilities. A normal person simply decides to go out to the corner to catch a bus or buy a paper. A disabled person probes the situation, asks whether it is feasible to even try to get to the corner, and if it is, by what means. And if I can get to the corner, why not try to reach the next corner, as well? What am I capable of? I will find out only by pressing on into the depth of body and spirit until I reach the point where I meet resistance. At that point of resistance, my body and spirit reveal stories to me, and in and through the particularities of those stories, I learn the truth about myself. In a poem called "Luca Signorelli's Resurrection of the Body," Jorie Graham

---

8. Birkerts, "Emerson's 'The Poet,'" 69.

tells the story of a fifteenth-century painter, who in his work sought to reveal the truth of the human body. But as the poet gazes upon the murals in a parish church, she realizes that: "*the wall / of the flesh / opens endlessly . . . .*"[9] So endlessly, in fact, that he could not find the point where it stopped and offered resistance to his probing.

Luca Signorelli was so frustrated by this endless opening of nature that when his only son died a violent death, the poem goes on, he had the corpse placed in his studio, where he cut (whether literally or figuratively the poet leaves to our interpretation) so deeply for so long that finally "his mind / could climb into // the open flesh and mend itself."[10] I may never reach the final resistance point where my reality is fully unveiled, but the probing (and caressing) is a truthing process. It is the way my mind climbs into the open flesh of my body's reality and there finds both truth and healing.

I must probe the world around me, as well, to see where it resists me. Much of the time, I feel as if the world is not made for disabled people—or for the disabled of any other species, for that matter. The natural order, and the social order, as well, favors those who can move around effortlessly. This means that in our efforts to enable the disabled, including the efforts of disabled persons themselves, we are going against the grain of evolutionary natural selection—all of our medical practice aims at the same thing, to foil the processes of natural selection. The very fact that such efforts require intense levels of imagination, expertise, technological resources, large sums of money, and vast expenditures of physical energy should remind us that we are contesting the structures bequeathed to us by the evolutionary process with counter-evolutionary means of our own devising. Why do we undertake such projects? As a disabled person, I live on the cusp of this evolution/counter-evolution interface, which fosters the sense of a lack of fit between me and the world, frequently in experiences that may seem small to most people. Get myself downtown to a building that is previously unknown to me and go to the entrance, only to find the sign "handicapped entrance around the corner." Ask for the key to a restroom, only to discover that the heavy door requires both hands to work the key in addition to a hearty push. Entire essays could be written on the theme, "Encountering doors." Since doors are entrances, they can symbolize how frustrating it

---

9. Graham, "Luca Signorelli's Resurrection," lines 68–70 pp. 76–77; also online: "Luca Signorelli's Resurrection," lines 68–70.

10. Graham, "Luca Signorelli's Resurrection," lines 103–106, p. 77; also online: "Luca Signorelli's Resurrection," lines 103–106.

is for a broken body simply to get in where it seeks to go. Many fine (and not so fine) restaurants place their tables so close together that a walker or a wheelchair or a wobbly cane-user can't get to a vacant chair. Theaters, opera houses, and ball parks can be a terror—only the expensive seats are handicapped friendly, forget the upper balcony, or even the lower. And busy people: it is quite understandable that a person who has only five minutes to get to a meeting—or is already late—will not hold the elevator for someone who is handicapped and slow moving. The most gracious host or hostess may live in a house or third floor walk-up that is virtually inaccessible to the handicapped. Small items they may be, but nevertheless they prompt the feeling that "I just don't belong here!" Audacity is essential to push back against this resistance of the world in order to discover what is possible. The university club I have enjoyed for many years has a grand staircase to the second floor dining room, but no proper elevator. An alert and kind maintenance man will commandeer the freight elevator that transports cartons and cans upstairs to the kitchen—I learned that I can cut quite a figure in dress suit and necktie riding amidst those crates and making my grand entrance through the kitchen to the banquet room! Female companions in stiletto heels and fine dresses may not get the same pleasure riding up next to a crate of canned tomatoes. Victories, some small, some large, may be difficult, but they regularly occur, and the disabled depend on them.

My spirit engages fully in this pressing to the point where I meet resistance—resistance from my own body and from the world around me. At every moment in this spiriting activity, the Spirit of God is engaging me.

I know of no more incisive description of this engagement of human spirit and God's Spirit than Saint Paul's words in the eighth chapter of Romans.

> You did not receive the spirit of slavery to fall back into fear, but you have received the spirit of sons and daughters. When we cry, "Abba! Father!" it is the Spirit itself bearing witness with our spirit that we are children of God, and if children, than heirs, heirs of God and fellow heirs of Christ, provided we suffer with him in order that we may also be glorified with him. . . . We know that the whole creation has been groaning in travail together until now; and not only the creation, but we ourselves, who have the first fruits of the Spirit, groan inwardly as we wait for adoption as sons and daughters, the redemption of our bodies. (Rom 8:15–17, 22–23)

Theologian Paul Tillich elaborated on Paul with his idea of "the manifestation of the divine Spirit in the human spirit." He writes that we "are conscious of being determined in [our] nature by spirit as a dimension of life."[11] Tillich understands that when our human spirit is engaged by God's Spirit, we are "driven into a successful self-transcendence." Our human spirit "remains what it is, but at the same time, it goes out of itself."[12] This going out of itself is termed "ecstasy."

I interpret my body's spiriting—as I have described the relentless pressing to discover what it is that my body exists for and what its possibilities are—as God's Spirit in terms that resonate, as well:

> All around us, to the right and left, in front and behind, above and below, we have only had to go a little beyond the frontier of sensible appearances in order to see the divine welling up and showing through.... It has sprung up so universally, and we find ourselves so surrounded and transfixed by it, that there is no room left to fall down and adore it, even within ourselves. By means of all created things, without exception, the divine assails us, penetrates us and molds us. We imagined it as distant and inaccessible, whereas in fact we live steeped in its burning layers.[13]

The body that is me remains what it is, but the ecstasy, the going out of itself is real and urgent. It is the constant questioning: What can I be? What should I do? Disabled persons know full well that these questions are the challenges to get out of ourselves—to submit to ecstasy. The alternative is despair, giving up that ecstasy is even a possibility and settling for the life of the scurrying ant!

Paul reminds me that if my body is a vessel of God's presence, the vessel is indeed an earthen one, just as Luther understood what every disabled person has to learn: God is hidden, even in the confines of my body. God's knitting of my body does not present a straight-forward beautiful pattern; there's an irony, even an absurdity, about these images—the same irony that attends the birth of Isaac, born when his parents, Abraham and Sarah, were in their nineties. We affirm that Mary's baby Jesus, born in obscurity, is the Incarnate Word of God, that ordinary bread can be the Eucharistic means of grace—also in their own way ironic statements of faith. Without transformation and a leap of faith, I could not ascribe God's presence to

---

11. Tillich, *Systematic Theology*, 3:111.
12. Ibid., 3:112.
13. Chardin, *Divine Milieu*, 112.

any of these events, let alone my own defective body. Tillich insisted that the Spirit of God is present in the midst of ambiguity, a lesson that disabled persons know with special clarity. In that ambiguity comes the cry to move in whatever way is possible and to be the more that our bodies can become.

In this, the disabled are Everyman and Everywoman, an epitome of what it means to be human. Disability may intensify universal human experience. Even though the awareness may not be so vivid, our bodies are bottom line for us all. For the able-bodied, spirit may seem to fly so high that body is inconsequential—this is not true for anyone, and for the disabled *denial of body is impossible*. Stereotypes that apply to most bodies hold less appeal to those who are focused simply on getting around, regardless of shape or sexual attractiveness and whether or not the lines of age are showing. Botox and breast enhancement cannot be top priority for those who are struggling to discern whether they can get around in any significant way. The stereotypes that are most destructive are those that depict the disabled as broken people who need repair or as a population that really doesn't matter.

The soul's desire for immortality animates us all; we feel it in our quest to overcome disease, our dreams of extending the span of our lives, our researching the magic of stem cells, and in our engineering fetuses and newborn babes. The same desire drives exploration of outer space and cyber space. It is the force behind the protest of the people of the underclass around the world who insist that they really do matter. Social disablement and physical handicap may indeed share a common dependence on the prodding of the spirit to press on through resistance to reach the promise of possibility.

God is present in all of these struggles, always hidden from ordinary discernment in ambiguity. Everyone who persists knows the irony of the situation in which we are placed. Essayist Sven Birkerts also wrote that his soul is "the part of the 'I' that recognizes the absurd fact of its being." Such recognition has not escaped the disabled. We know that the danger lurks in despair and cynicism that would deny that possibility is real.

I said earlier that disability has revealed to me how deeply and utterly dependent I am, on a network of technology and other people. Deeper still is my dependence on the Spirit of God that keeps my soul alive. This, I share with all of God's people everywhere.

To the Knitter
(August 10, 2012)

Shit!
this is your
idea of a sweater
your
design
of a body

You didn't tell me
that it would
begin
unraveling
at precisely
the place
you started
dropping stitches

This is your great idea
of a
body

Yes, I know
that I got
better than
I deserve
and what's left
works better than
ever can be justified
at four score,
But still—
is
whirlwind speech
all I get
in explanation
My protest is
not Job's
nor Lear's

Our Bodies Are Selves

What would you expect
mine is what
a prissy
watered down
american christian
can muster—
an insult to
you
and
me

pathos—
where I had hoped
for tragedy
is this
your design
too

3

Personal Narrative
Living in the Middle Years

Ann Milliken Pederson

Such sensations make me think of my girlhood. I look closely at each memory, in my own gallery, as if to discover some clue, some fresh element in the story: a hand on an arm, a glove left on an arm, a glance, a glove left on a seat, maybe.[1]

MEMORIES CAN BE LIKE paintings in a gallery that we can stroll through, gazing at them and then pausing to examine the details. Or memories can come and go, unexpectedly; they interrupt us in the middle of our story. Suddenly, scenes send us reeling into our past. I can feel those memories in my body when I think about why my knees bother me now almost forty years later from carrying forty-five pound packs up trails in the mountains. Or the tenderness I sense in my hands whenever I try to practice the piano but can't because of too many years at the computer. But I am also grateful that now at the age of fifty-six, I still have a bodyself that carries the genes of family members who often live into their nineties, and not just "live," but

---

1. Chessman, *Lydia Cassatt Reading*, 23.

live well. My uncle remarked how tired he was from dancing the night away at a charity ball the other night. He is ninety-two years old. My gallery of memories is rich indeed.

One memory I have is from a scene at a local cafe. My husband and I gather with friends on a rather regular basis to share a meal—companions, literally, eating bread together. On this intensely warm, if not hot, late September evening, we met at Parker's, a downtown bistro. Whenever we all eat at this small, exquisite place, I find myself thinking about the final scenes in *Babette's Feast,* a movie that embodies what I hope the final feast will be.[2] The meal that is prepared by Babette, the French gourmand, draws together and transforms the elderly villagers who live in a remote province of Denmark called Jutland. They come as elders, their bodies betraying the toll of the years of living together in harsh climates and in a closely knit community where they knew each other's business all too well. Grudges were kept for decades and village gossip turned into epic stories. But then they gather for a meal, lavishly, extravagantly, and lovingly prepared. These quarrelsome villagers leave the meal transformed, becoming friends and companions again, filled with a renewed vigor and passion for life ahead, whatever it may be.

While the meal I ate with my friends is hardly on par with the great artistic canvas painted in *Babette's Feast,* I find that after Gary and I leave the restaurant we, too, are transformed from the middle-aged-almost-now-senior citizens that we have become into individuals with a renewed passion and zest for life. We try not to talk about the toll that age has taken on our bodies, our memories, indeed, ourselves. But that is our reality. We are in the middle of our lives, moving into the later years. This is the point from which I will reflect on what it means to know who I am as a bodyself. The struggle, of course, is trying to find an adequate vocabulary to speak about how we know who we are and what we think it means to be embodied. I find that the expressions of what it means to share meals with companions serves me well—a sacramental vocabulary of words turning into flesh. The Word becomes words only when we can smell, see, touch, taste, and hear. My own Lutheran sensibility, refined by years of visiting and living with my Roman Catholic relatives, shapes how I know my bodyself. The rhythms of the liturgical year, the prayers of the daily offices, and the sacramental moments of Baptism and Eucharist inform and shape what it means to be a bodyself and to be part of the body of God.

2. *Babette's Feast.*

These expressions of friendship are sacrament for me—moments where the metaphysical nature of friendship is transformed into little Eucharists—foretastes of feasts yet to come. I begin where I am—in these middle years, knowing that while much of my life has past, I have much in my future for which I am already grateful. I offer these reflections on the liturgical year and daily offices as a way into knowing what it means for me to be a bodyself.

IN THE MIDDLE OF BEGINNINGS: ADVENT AND MATINS

> We give thanks to you, heavenly Father, through Jesus Christ your dear Son, that you have protected us through the night from all danger and harm. We ask you to preserve and keep us, this day also, from all sin and evil, that in all our thoughts, words, and deeds we may serve and please you. Into your hands we commend our bodies and souls and all that is ours. Let your holy angels have charge of us, that the wicked one have no power over us.[3]

This prayer was Luther's Morning Prayer. How appropriate—its baptismal imagery of dying and rising anew each day reminds us of our beginnings, of our origins in God. Baptism is my beginning: October 6, 1957 to be exact. This spiritual commencement was my entrance into the family of God. I love the beginning of a new year and a new day. I'm always relieved when I get up from bed, and realize that I'm alive, awake, and that each day is a new start. This prayer from Matins reminds me that every moment is a gift. September ushers in another new beginning when the opening of the academic year arrives, and I can feel the change from the heat of the summer to the cool of the fall. Advent opens the liturgical year of the Christian church. During those cold, December interludes, the shadows lengthen and the evening arrives sooner, signaling the end of the busyness of the day.

The First Sunday in Advent is my favorite beginning of a new year. This Sunday marks another beginning of the year—the liturgical year of the Christian church. Christ the King Sunday, with its strange royal imagery, is gone. Fall is gone. Winter is here today, with the first new snowfall. The shadows are falling at the day's end—much earlier. Time is a strange passage. We mark passages of our lives by events: birthdays, anniversaries,

---

3. "Prayer at the Close of the Day," *ELW* 163.

and deaths. A friend of mine told me that she waits anxiously when all her synchronized clocks turn 11:11 am or pm—all those 1s in a row. We know what time it is when our stomachs growl or when we can't stay awake during the 10 pm news (that's just old age, some would say). The rhythms of our bodies beat, contract, breathe—autosomatically. Tornado sirens warn of pending storms and church bells welcome people to worship. Generations of families pass by and geological eras cut through the landscape. In South Dakota we joke that we have two seasons: road construction and potholes. We can instantly message our friends through cyberspace. We wait in the doctors' office for test results, and all of a sudden time comes to a halt. As I write this, it's Advent, waiting season again.

The beginning of the church year is like the beginning of each day—promises that God will be waiting for us and with us. "Morning Has Broken" is one of my favorite hymns.[4] Creation is a beginning, and it begins anew each day. Every day is a reenactment of God's recreating work. With creation, however, also comes destruction and with the brilliance of new life arrives the loss in death. Humans arrived on the planet as a result of millions of other species dying. Beginnings and endings are built into the way we take in the world through our bodyselves. To start my mornings, I look out the patio doors, waiting for the arrival of the birds to the feeders. I know the black-capped chickadee, the nuthatch, the downy woodpecker, the pair of cardinals, lots and lots of sparrows, and maybe a flycatcher. The sparrows come in groups of ten to twenty, nibble at the feeders and they fly away as quickly as they came. The woodpecker heads right to the suet and often hangs upside down or parallel to the feeder. The male's bright red head offsets the black and white patterned body.

Byron and Jack, my companion species, also look out the patio windows. They are much less interested in the birds, but eagerly await the arrival of the squirrel. If I'm in another room, I know the squirrel is sitting atop the feeder because I can hear the loud barking that ensues. While I wait to watch the birds, enjoying their morning feedings, Byron and Jack await the squirrel, hoping that I'll let them out in time to have their own kind of morning "feeding." One time my friend called me and told me that her dog had caught a squirrel and was in the process of digesting it—she told me every part that went down that Labrador's mouth. But somehow I always feel a bit sorry for the squirrel and give it a quick warning to flee before I let the dogs dash out madly after the squirrel: prey and predator.

---

4. Eleanor Farjeon, "Morning Has Broken," hymn 556.

However, sometimes the squirrel runs up the tree and then chatters loudly, teasing and harassing the poodle.

Different views through my patio windows remind me that nature is not just a pastoral picture of beauty. Nature is also "red in tooth and claw."[5] That is one view. But alongside this view is that of another poet, "And for all this, nature is never spent. There lives the dearest freshness deep down things,"[6] who also reminds me that God broods over the world with, "Ah, bright wings."[7] These two views through my patio window belong to the same world, and are created by the same God.

With beginnings come endings. I just met a young woman who is helping me to know what it's like to begin again when something has come to an end. Several years ago she had a brain tumor removed; she had cancer. And when the tumor was gone, so was much of her memory. And now years later, she stills struggles with details that I realize are second nature to me. It's like someone telling you that you once knew how to ride a bike but now, all of a sudden, you can't remember how. You can't remember where the pedals are, or how to steer. The kinesthetic memories sometimes are beyond her grasp.

She describes to me moments where she knows she knows something: she feels it but when she tries to find the language to describe those feelings and thoughts, the words are submerged. I'm trying to imagine what it would be like to learn again, to begin again and again, over and over with the same things. The closest thing I can relate to is when I have tried to learn a new language. It just takes practice, lots and lots of practice. When I'm finally dreaming in that language, then I know that I *know* the language. When I was studying Greek at the seminary, I would get up and realize that I had been thinking in Greek. The words were still vivid in those waking moments. It had become second nature to me. The challenge for both of us, my student and me, is realizing how difficult it is to begin again when something has come to an end. That which was second nature now must become a new labor of love.

We know our beginnings by those who have gone before us, our ancestors whose lives are now only memories. But those recollections are often like those of this student that I have met; they are not just "out there" somewhere, as if in a disembodied place; they are in our cells, genes, and

---

5. Alfred Lord Tennyson, "In Memoriam A. H. H.," canto LVI, line 15.
6. Gerard Manley Hopkins, "God's Grandeur," lines 9–10.
7. Ibid., line 14.

tissues. Learning about my ancestry, about those who have gone before me, is profoundly spiritual and deeply sensual. I have traveled with my mother to Sharon, North Dakota, and her birthplace. The family legend is that she was born during a blizzard in the back of a building that housed the bowling alley. A town that once had a post office, a couple of churches, railway station, and grocery store, is now nearly empty. The census records show that eighty-two people now populate Sharon. Someday the little North Dakota town might be gone. Only the graves in the nearby cemetery will help me remember where my mother's family came from. I don't remember her mother—she died of breast cancer when I was two. I know that breast cancer is a part of my ancestry, a reminder of what it means to be female in my family. Our bodies carry inside of us the trauma of our origins.

I will always carry within me the trauma of a sexual assault that occurred much earlier in my life. For years afterward, I was afraid—of men, of walking on the streets alone, of going to sleep at night and worrying about what my dreams might be. But I have learned that even this event cannot and will not define my true origins. I am more than a survivor; I have learned to live again. My baptism reminds me that nothing can separate me from God's love, that no trauma will mark my life forever. Instead, the mark of the cross on my forehead and chest, given to me at Baptism, is the mark of new beginnings. Nothing can separate me from God's love. That is what it means to have a beginning, to know my origins as a child of God.

IN THE MIDDLE OF THE DAYS: SUFFRAGES AND AN AFTERNOON PRAYER

> O God, in you we live and move and have our being. Guide and govern us in this day by your Holy Spirit, that in all the cares and occupations of our life we may not forget you, but remember that always we are walking in your sight; through Jesus Christ our Lord.[8]

At our neighboring Lutheran church, the front of the sanctuary has a painted mosaic of the ascension. Jesus is rising into the sky, while his beloved disciples gaze from below. In the mosaic, Jesus has neither fully left the ground, nor fully risen into the heights of heaven. This picture so often represents my life. It is an image that is familiar to us—we are not fully

---

8. "Responsive Prayer," 330.

grounded in the moment. We are on the way somewhere. Here, not there. I am still here, grounded so to speak, but not really. I think about that list that reminds me of what I must yet do and don't really want to do—the piles of laundry waiting to be washed and ironed, the floors that need another quick attack by the vacuum, and all the papers that need to be graded. To be or not to be is the refrain of my lists. I'm haunted by that refrain. I want to *be*—fully present in the moment; not always caught somewhere in between. I teach college students and they are the ultimate embodiment of this living in between—they wait for acceptance to medical school, for the job interview, for summer camp to begin, for a wedding. Life is lived in the middle—between past and present, between here and there. Somehow I must find a way to live in between, *in medias res*, without falling behind or racing ahead of myself. I have decided that the festival of the Ascension, which celebrates Jesus' departure from earth, is one in which the church understands this experience of living in between.

Life is always in-between: between what we love so dearly, and want to cling to, from our past and what we long for in the future. But the power and grace of the moment slips away from us. This living in between creates a kind of ongoing anxiety, uncertainty, and frustration. I know how those lists haunt the dreams in my restless nights, or create the pounding in my heart when I know I am racing to catch up once again. The now and the not yet—what do I do with my life? What do I long for? This question has become more urgent as the years slip by more quickly, each one of them a testament to my age.

What it is that I crave, that I long for so deeply? To find food that will "satisfy the hungry heart."[9] However, our fast-paced, consumer driven culture advertises on my television, computer, and phone that these needs can be met quickly, and to my satisfaction. Rarely, however, does that happen. We seem to crave that which satisfies us easily and quickly. Fastfood chains are a way of life for many of us as we pass on our way to other parts of our lives. My husband will attest to my love of Egg McMuffins or a tasty supper of Spaghetti Os and canned peas. We learned early in our marriage which of the two of us is the better cook. Now that high blood pressure and extra pounds define my midlife body, I must find other, more healthful ways to take care of my bodyself. It's not easy. The patterns I have established and fall back on almost every day are not easy to give up because they are so familiar and comfortable. They work for the time being. But now even those

9. Westendorff, "You Satisfy the Hungry Heart," hymn 484.

midnight forages in the freezer don't work anymore. After a steady diet of unhealthy foods, I become even more voracious for that which really satisfies. I am full, but always empty.

What is it that I crave, that I long for? This fall I reread Michael Pollan's book, *The Botany of Desire* and Barbara Kingsolver's *Animal, Vegetable, Miracle*.[10] The authors challenge my desire for a quick fix and almost provoked me to grow my own food and cook our household meals. But I know better so I continue to assign the preparation of our food to my husband. I did indulge in one new habit this fall that I intend to make an annual one. On several occasions we drove to local apple orchards and picked our own from the trees. While I was hardly in the Garden of Eden, the experience was a close approximation. I loved reaching overhead to pull the ripening Honeycrisps from the branches. Better yet was the experience of eating them for weeks afterwards. They tasted like nothing I had eaten from the store. I can see why Eve was tempted.

We try to fill our own physical and spiritual needs. We can never have enough. I ask my friends who are cleaning out a house before moving into a new one and they always tell me that they have more than enough stuff. Garage sale signs are abundant in our neighborhoods. We have trouble distinguishing our needs from our desires. However, I know that the luxury of having way too much or even just enough is not the reality of many who live in the world, in Sioux Falls, South Dakota, and even in my neighborhood. One in six children still suffer from poverty, and probably go hungry at night. I don't think I have any idea how easy I really have it. When I take in much more than I can actually eat, I get indigestion. Antacids are a staple of my diet. My restlessness in life betrays my impatience with it. I still try to fill my deep, spiritual longings with the fast food of life, with the McDonald's hamburgers that give us immediate satisfaction; however, the food that Jesus offers is different. It satisfies my deepest longings, and there are baskets left over for others. Can I take in the food that God gives us? What exactly am I hungry for? Helping to fill the hunger of others will lead me to satisfying my own hungry heart.

I should recite this prayer each day:

> We give thanks to you, heavenly Father, through Jesus Christ your dear Son, that you have protected us through the night from all danger and harm. We ask you to preserve and keep us, this day also, from all sin and evil, that in all our thoughts, words, and

---

10. Pollan, *Botany of Desire* (2002); Kingsolver, *Animal, Vegetable, Miracle* (2008).

> deeds we may serve and please you. Into your hands we commend our bodies and souls and all that is ours. Let your holy angels have charge of us, that the wicked one have no power over us.[11]

These words become food not only for thought, but also for my body. The sacrament of the present moment of prayer is to let God receive my anxieties, tensions, and uncertainties, and transform me so that I am living fully in the presence of God's grace. The words of this prayer become grace notes that free me to live fully and fruitfully in the sacrament of the present moment. Don't cling to the past, or worry about the future—I am called to live in between, in the present moment of God's loving grace.

AT THE END OF OUR DAYS: FROM VESPERS TO COMPLINE

> O God, you have called your servants to ventures of which we cannot see the ending, by paths as yet untrodden, through perils unknown. Give us faith to go out with good courage, not knowing where we go, but only that your hand is leading us and your love supporting us; through Jesus Christ our Lord.[12]

The prayer from Vespers reminds us that we are on a lifelong journey. The prayer from Compline reminds us that we dwell in God's peace. I can feel this tension expressed in my body—I'm on a quest to know why, but at the same time I long to dwell in God's peace. Such tension resides in the questions we ask and in the tragedies we experience that make no sense at all. Last year one of Gary's middle school band students was killed in a fire in her own home. Three of the children didn't make it and the mother was eventually charged with possession of controlled substances and child neglect. She wasn't home at the time of the fire. I remember the girl, Shannon, who carried her baritone in the fall parade where the middle school band had its first marching event. When our friends met Gary and the kids at the end of the parade route, there was no one to pick her up. She had to walk the mile home, carrying her horn, and would probably arrive at an empty house. Gary traded her horn for a jacket that some kid had left and we walked with her up Phillips Avenue where the parade had been.

---

11. "Responsive Prayer," *ELW*, 330.
12. "Evening Prayer," *ELW*, 317.

We were astonished when later in the year Gary received news from the other band director that the kids had been killed in the fire. I couldn't get her face out of my head and I still remember her. I have no idea where God is in the details of these incidents. But we are called to remember and to travel the journey to bring some meaning to the disaster. God is hidden and revealed in the memories, questions, and the calls for help. I have no comforting resolution to this story.

I am grateful simply for the prayers of Vespers and Compline. I can say them with the generations before me who also had no answers, but gathered together in prayer. We will rarely see an ending, a result. We don't know where we're going because the question itself will not have an ending, and could be fraught with dangers, and may include many detours. The only thing we seem to know from this prayer is that God goes with us. That is my hope. We know that God's hand is with us and God's love is with us. In a way that's an answer to the question. Maybe our venture in the world is to ask the questions knowing that we won't find an answer and that the journey could be a long and dangerous one. For some, the question may lead to letting go of God's hand. For others, God's hand may lead directly into God's world and we will find ourselves along the way asking the question with millions of other pilgrims through the centuries. Or we might find ourselves in the middle of our own lives, finding other people that need our help, support, and love. That's why I love reading the work of theologian Dietrich Bonhoeffer. He finds God in the *midst* of the world. Not at the edges where we've shoved God when there are no answers, but in the middle of life's beginnings and endings.

When a friend asked me what one of my favorite books that I read was, I have answered, *Body of Work* by Christine Montross. After I tell her that the book is about a medical student's relationship with her cadaver that she dissects, the conversation comes to a dead halt. Why would someone who is not a healthcare professional or scientist want to read a book about cadavers? Christine Montross writes: "The dead body harbors the great mysteries of creation and humanity . . . ."[13] Death reveals life. One time when I told someone I was preaching on Ash Wednesday, she recalled the times she has had ashes put on her forehead. She replied, "Someday I'm going to say—You are dust and to dust you shall return. So, deal with it." We are creatures, mortal and finite. All humans share the same "condition," and it is primary, progressive, and terminal. We are mortal. No one is exempt

13. Montross, *Body of Work*, 2.

from being human. All of us die. I recognize this in ways that have been profoundly painful, but also marvelously transformative.

Along with reading a morbid book about cadavers, I have also watched a movie that has now become one of my favorites. Again, the subject is bodies and death. *Departures* is about a young man whose job is preparing bodies of the dead before they are placed in the coffin and eventually cremated.[14] What starts as a job turns into a vocation, and he becomes an artist at taking care of and working with the dead and the families who grieve for their loved ones. By the end of the film I was left with a deep appreciation of life by watching how someone respected and took care of those who died. Death ushers in life and endings become beginnings. I have never been so deeply and profoundly moved by a movie.

I know when I feel alive: when I'm in love with what I do and with the people around me. This does not mean the tasks or the relationships are easy. More often than not the opposite is the case. My good friend LuAnn, who is a palliative care physician, says that most of us as we age will become more and more like who we are now, in our middle years. We will die as we have lived. One of my greatest fears is that I will die without knowing that which makes me come alive, that which is given to me by God. When I counsel students about their futures, I tell them to try and do what they love. They will find their vocation in that love. When I am most fully alive is when I'm engaged most deeply with others around me, albeit human or non-human. And yet much of that which surrounds me works to create the opposite—a kind of deadness, or apathy. My bodyself knows how to do more and more, faster and faster. But I also know that this is not life-giving.

So many of us are always looking ahead for something new or in other cases worrying about what's happened in the past. And consequently the joy of the present moment is gone. Instead of living through instant messages, we should take time to know someone in person. We can take in the bigger picture, and relish the longer time frame. Our bodyselves might learn to relax, and not simply multi-task the day away. More and more research shows that multi-tasking doesn't accomplish more; it just creates busy, tired people who don't do anything very well. Paying attention is cultivating the habit of knowing where we are at this moment in time.

From graduate school through tenure as a college professor, I have bought into the all-American sport of competing as a top-notch workaholic. Many days I could win a gold medal. But the spiritual problem is

---

14. *Departures* (2008).

still the same: thinking that my worth and wholeness as a human being is dependent solely on what others think of me, of living up to someone else's standards. Like the constricting pilgrimages and programs of penance in the sixteenth century, I had found ways to produce more, do more, and in such a way that it only enhanced my anxiety and exhaustion. Last spring I went to my internal medicine doctor with the problem of recurring, severe headaches. The diagnosis was "that I worked too much." She said to me: "What do you expect me to do about this? I can't just prescribe pills, you know. It seems to me that you have to want to be well, to feel good, and that means you need to change." So, instead of pain killers, I was given a prescription for physical therapy. I have encountered a new reformer who I doubt would have thought of himself as such.

Little did I know that what began as weekly massages and the deep heat of ultrasound would give way to rigorous and exhausting routines on the "reformer," the machine developed by Joseph Pilates. Now, two months into my Pilates regimen I have learned through practice and hard work how to relax, to let go, to breathe more deeply.

Joseph Pilates was born in Germany in 1880 to a mother of German descent and a father from Greece.[15] From his father he inherited the love of gymnastics and from his mother, the knowledge of her naturopathic medicine. As an unhealthy child, he struggled to overcome his physical weakness and began studying and practicing body building and gymnastics to strengthen his body. During World War I, he was stationed in a camp in England with other German inmates. There he began to teach them exercise and strengthening techniques. When he returned to Germany, he developed machines and exercises to help soldiers rehabilitate their bodies from the trauma of the war. One such machine (still in use by those who practice Pilates) is called the reformer. Adapted from his work in hospital units, the machine uses springs and sliding platforms. Joseph Pilates used the equipment available to him at the patients' bedsides in order to develop his programs of exercise and rehabilitation.

Joseph Pilates came to believe that the "modern" lifestyle of his time and its symptomatic embodiments were the problem of sickness and anxiety. For example, he thought that shallow breathing symbolized someone's inability to keep up with the frenetic pace of their life. When stress takes over one's life, one's breathing becomes more staccato and fast-paced. The shallow breathing often accompanies poor posture and an anxious spirit.

---

15. Pilates Foundation, "History of Pilates;" Keene, "Pilates, Joseph Hubertus."

Seeking to change the people embodied by these unhealthy cultural ways of life, Joseph Pilates became a reformer of mind and body. His method of exercise became famous and was soon adopted by dancers (like Martha Graham) and today has become one of the most popular ways to strengthen the body and increase flexibility.

I remember in the 1980s when Jane Fonda's workout routine first came on the market. A friend and I would don our leotards and work for the "burn" that Fonda insisted was a sign of good exercise. The burn that one felt deep in the muscles was usually preceded by fast-paced, often frantic repetitions. Ironically, such exercise seemed to mirror the spirit of that decade. While I no doubt had flatter abs and stronger leg muscles, I did not have a calmer spirit. The exercise matched my personal aspirations: to do more, and to do it better.

After a decade of frantic Fonda, new ways of exercising have taken its place. Yoga and Pilates are popular for different reasons than Fonda's workout. Instead of doing more and more at a faster and faster pace, these exercise disciplines (and in the case of yoga, spiritual as well) emphasize pacing one's self, breathing deeply, and centering one's body. Pilates practices the following principles: proper alignment of the spine, paying deep attention to the movements, slow and careful breathing, graceful and flowing movements, concentration, and control. Pilates can become a new style of life where the crazy pace of modern culture is counter-embodied with grace, breath, strength, and flexibility.

When I first started Pilates as part of a physical therapy regiment, I had no idea what to expect. Nicole, my physical therapist, began to teach me how to breathe, deeply through my diaphragm and out slowly through my mouth. While I had been taught this earlier in my life when learning to play the flute, I had never thought of this deep breathing technique as the way I should always breathe. All the time, breathing deeply, inhaling into my rib cage, and exhaling just as fully. All of the Pilates exercises rely on this breathing technique. From learning how to breathe again, I moved on to the mat routine, which involves focusing on one's core area. I had no idea how difficult this would be.

Nicole is not only a physical therapist, but also a high school soccer coach. She wore both hats as my new Pilates trainer. She was gentle with me, but persistent, always insisting that I could do a bit more. When I left those sessions with her, my body felt a new kind of exhaustion. Not the burn of Fonda days, but the total collapse of a deep fatigue. Little things started to change. I began to sleep better, be more alert during the day, and walk with more confidence. Slowly, my body has trained my mind, and lifted my spirit. Or possibly for the first time in a long while, I am a whole person—body/mind/spirit is as one. In fact, the delight I have found in practicing Pilates is that my muscles teach my mind and spirit. So often I have lived with the opposite notion—that I could think my way into relaxing. Pilates joins the mind and spirit to the body's graceful, slow movements. My muscles and lungs teach me, nurture me, and remind me that strength develops over time, and that grace is a gift that is learned. Breathing deeply counteracts the fast-pace of American culture. We are created in the image of God as a counter reflection of what our culture expects us to be. To reflect on God's image is to discover what it means to truly be free, to love and accept who we are because we are already loved and accepted by God. We can let go of the cultural idols that enslave our bodyselves and be free for others.

Death can come at once, or slowly and incrementally over a lifespan. My hope is that I will always ask and do what makes me come alive. When I smell pine trees, or read a novel by my favorite author, or learn something new with college students, or hold a dying person's hand, I know that my life is meeting the needs of others. If we simply live by asking what others want and need, we ignore that which God has given us. And that which we are given comes by surprise, in unexpected ways. That's one definition of grace. If indeed I am created by God as a creature that means I'm both finite and mortal.

As I age, I'm more and more aware of my limits. I have a new wonder about life, and yet it is always accompanied by a sense of loss—that I will never have again the day that I have just lived. I am simultaneously hopeful and awe struck about the mystery of life and yet deeply saddened by how abruptly the lives of those I love come to an end. The boundaries between life and death are elusive—the fleeting markers of what makes us human. Birth and death seem less like the terminal points we think they are and more like fleeting moments in a great cosmic dance.

As I grow older, my perspective has changed. Beginnings and endings can be abrupt departures and take offs, like the moments we lurch on and off the runways. My life is terminal, at least this life I know on this earth. And the rhythms of life and death, evening and morning of a new day, mark the way I live. Martin Luther knew this so deeply and he reminded Christians like me to mark myself with the sign of the cross every morning and evening. We are to remember who we are and whose we are, and even where we are going. Matins, Prayer at Midday, Vespers, and Compline have marked the church days and years for centuries. They mark my daily life, when I remember. I live by the rhythms of beginnings and endings, dying and rising to new days and new years. So, I know that I must live in between the beginnings and endings with a purpose and passion that honors the day God has given me.

COMPLINE: PRAYER AT THE CLOSE OF THE DAY

O Lord, support us all the day long of this troubled life, until the shadows lengthen and the evening comes and the busy world is hushed, the fever of life is over, and our work is done. Then, Lord, in your mercy, grant us a safe lodging, and a holy rest, and peace at the last; through Jesus Christ our Lord.[16]

---

16. "Night Prayer," *ELW*, 325.

4

In the Early Years
Tiny Promises

Susan Barreto

from the mother's womb
Untimely born

ADAPTED FROM SHAKESPEARE *MACBETH* 5.10.14–16

ONE EARLY FROSTY SATURDAY morning in mid-December, one mom and dad were initially told that there was a 25 percent chance that their third child, a newborn baby girl, would live. This was simply due to the fact that she was born in 1973, happened to weigh 2 pounds 1 ounce, was born weeks early, and was in a hospital in rural Northwestern Illinois. Quickly realizing the situation's seriousness, a local pediatrician suggested transporting the baby to the nearest state-run hospital with a preemie center in Peoria, Illinois.

If the statistics would have been bleaker, there would have been little need to heed the doctor's advice, but my parents made the painful decision to let me spend the first months of my life in a neonatal intensive care unit that they knew nothing about roughly 120 miles away. The action likely saved my life, while at the time I'm sure it seemed to be a desperate measure. My mother wrote at the time, "Immediately following our discussion on hospital care, I was allowed to see Susan for the first time. My heart cried out as I looked through the glass walls of the incubator. I thought I had myself conditioned not to get attached to her, in case we lost her; but love swelled in my heart immediately. I thanked God for my daughter and for the love I felt for her. I learned love is never wasted, so let it flow."

I was transferred to St. Francis Hospital's Premature Station, which was one of the first specialized units of its kind in the country when it was set up in 1942. It housed all the most up-to-date medical equipment and provided excellent, around-the-clock care. I was fed initially intravenously through the veins in my scalp. I had a Styrofoam disc attached to my abdomen area that was a thermostat to keep the isolette at a constant temperature. There were also two tiny red electrodes attached to my chest to track my breath rate at all times. My mother recalls that a machine recorded it all.

To treat jaundice, an ultraviolet light shined over my body in the isolette. Thick bandages covered my eyes to protect them from the rays, while my hands were held down on either side by bands so that I couldn't reach the bandages, tubes, and other attachments.

My diapers were weighed to determine my nutrition. Sadly after two weeks, I hadn't gained an ounce. Most babies in the first month of life gain at least a few ounces, if not more, but in my case it took more than a month to do so. After sixty days I weighed in at a whopping 4 pounds 9 ounces, which was enough to allow me to go home. Early photos from those days were of me next to a glass Pepsi bottle that was longer than me!

Today, the St. Francis' NICU admits more than 650 newborns, and each year the care and technology of critically ill newborns improves. In addition to monitoring, respiratory therapy, and surgical expertise, the unit is also home to memorial services and hospice facilities. There are organizations that are dedicated to taking photos of babies not expected to make it. Now I Lay Me Down to Sleep employs volunteer photographers to take beautiful images of the baby and family that provide captivating images that are integral to helping the family heal after their loss, which is sometimes within hours of the photo session.[1] The remembrance photography is free to the grieving family.

---

1. www.nowilaymedowntosleep.org.

"On Saturday March 17, 2012, around 10:45 am, we said hello and good-bye to our beloved son," writes one family of their Now I Lay Me Down to Sleep experience.[2] "It is shocking to know that he is physically no longer with us. Yet we are glad that your organization exists and was able to provide us a lifetime of memories through the baby pictures taken of him. We are so grateful and thank God that we have these pictures to forever treasure our baby angel. May God continue to bless you as you bless and help families through their difficult time."

Premature infants born today at my birth size have a 90 percent survival rate. In fact, in a recent conversation with the father of a premature baby girl, he and his wife were very concerned, but had been given greater assurances for survival than my parents were. His biggest shock was the thousands of dollars in medical bills that were incurred as a result of the prolonged hospital stay and the fact that all the clothes passed down from an older sister had no way of fitting!

All that technology that continues to evolve to keep the tiniest among us alive is a miracle to behold. It certainly was the case as far back as the turn of the century when premature babies were on display at Coney Island. Yes, incubators were sold primarily to hospitals and amusement parks in the 1920s and 1930s! How did premature infants become a sideshow attraction? Dr. Martin A. Couney is said to have saved thousands of infants by putting incubators of prematurely born babies on display and the treatment of babies were paid for through the collection of 10 cents a piece by visitors.[3] Other prominent exhibits of preemies Dr. Couney set up included the 1933 World's Fair Exhibition in Chicago.[4]

Dr. Couney is credited with broadening the acceptance of the incubator in the United States. Born in Alsace, France, he was trained in Berlin. The "incubator doctor" began his work by displaying incubators developed by his mentors at the Berlin Exposition of 1896. After saving as many as 8,000 babies by some estimates, Dr. Couney died broken and forgotten in 1950 at eighty years old. He had the reputation of a shady sideshow showman, but had the medical acumen to do lifesaving work for families who would have lost their children if it weren't for the Coney Island exhibit.

---

2. Now I Lay Me Down to Sleep, "Family Testimonials," last par.

3. Oral History Archive: Voices from Coney Island, "Roslyn Tromer: Incubator Baby," first interview.

4. Brick, "And Next to the Bearded Lady."

These sideshow attractions must have sparked curiosity over how some of the smallest humans could survive through the help of technology. Today, though, are we in awe over the strength of the infants in the incubators or at ourselves for creating technology that can overcome almost certain death?

The human body has an amazing capacity for survival. Babies born at twenty-three weeks (just under six months along in the pregnancy) have a 17 percent chance of survival. Only two weeks later, a preemie's chances greatly improve to 50 percent. To be considered extremely low birth weight a baby weighs 2.2 pounds or less.[5] James Elgin Gill (born on May 20, 1987 in Ottawa, Canada) was the earliest premature baby in the world.[6] He was 128 days premature (twenty-one weeks and five days gestation) and weighed 1 pound 6 ounces. He survived. The record for the smallest premature baby to survive was held for some time by Madeline Mann, who was born at twenty-six weeks weighing 9.9 ounces and was 9.5 inches long.[7] But this record was broken in 2004 by Rumaisa Rahman, who was born in the same hospital at twenty-five weeks gestation.[8] At birth she was 8 inches long and weighed 8.6 ounces. Her twin sister was also a small baby, weighing 1 pound 4 ounces at birth.

As the babies surviving seem to get smaller, it is also worth noting that the percentage of preemie births has also risen in recent years, with nearly 13 percent of all live births being preterm in the US as of 2006, according to National Center for Health Statistics.[9] The Child Health Epidemiology Reference Group—an NGO that assists both WHO and UNICEF—estimates that 15 million preemies are born worldwide annually.[10]

While it cost less than fifteen dollars a day to keep a preemie at Coney Island in the 1930s and 40s,[11] today's medical bills add up quickly to thousands of dollars a day as the technology has improved to the point that the mortality rate has dropped dramatically over the last twenty plus years. The cost in the first few months may be sizable, but perhaps complicating

---

5. Quint Boenker Preemie Survival Foundation, "Preemie Survival."
6. CanWest News Service, "Miracle Child."
7. Prasad, "A Little Miracle."
8. Nanji, "World's Smallest Baby."
9. Martin, Joyce, et al. "Births: Final Data," 2.
10 Blencowe, "National, Regional, and Worldwide," 2167, further discussion at 2168–71.
11. Zahorsky, "Baby Incubators," 349.

matters further is the fact that while the ability to keep extremely premature babies alive continues to improve, those children are much more likely to have more lifelong complications and disabilities.

It is estimated that half the preemies born before the twenty-sixth week of gestation are disabled, according to a report cited on the website. In a 2009 meta-analysis of fourteen studies, researchers found that very preterm babies were likely to have moderate to severe deficits in academic achievement, attention problems, and internalizing behavioral problems.[12] These issues were strongly correlated to their immaturity at birth. The study said that during transition to young adulthood these children continue to be behind their full-term peers. Numerous studies have investigated the preemie situation from various angles to report findings such as preemies being at higher risk for depression and schizophrenia and that these babies are less likely to be fully engaged at the cognitive level by the time they reach school.

So what does all this cost society? In 2007, the Institute of Medicine tallied up that premature birth in the US alone cost $26.2 billion each year, most of which ($16.9 billion) was for medical costs related to the baby.[13] The US is unique though in that nearly 500,000 preemies are born here each year, which is the highest figure of any other industrialized country. Special education and early intervention services total more than $2 billion for children three to twenty-one years old. The mothers' medical bills total $1.9 billion, while another $5.7 billion is the cost in lost work and wages for people born prematurely.[14] The last figure is based off of the trend that in some instances premature birth can create long-term health conditions and disabilities that prevent them from working. Supplemental Security Income in the US pays benefits to disabled adults and children who have limited income and resources.

The sheer survivability and amazing tales of miraculous life in a tiny package has really changed the way Americans view premature babies. They are now patients to be cared for rather than objects of pity or of sideshow curiosity. While many programs continue to promote greater prenatal care and nutrition has generally improved over the last century, the littlest of the little ones are still with us.

---

12. Aarnoudse-Moens, "Meta-Analysis of Neurobehavioral Outcomes," 717–28.
13. Behrman and Butler, *Preterm Birth*, 399.
14. Ibid., 11, 47, 398–99, 425.

In the worst cases, these babies may have cerebral palsy or severe vision problems (as I myself have struggled with over the years).[15] They may even be reliant on oxygen tanks their entire lives.[16] As we have battled end-of-life questions for the elderly and the terminally ill, it begs the question of whether all the medical intervention for preemies leads to a quality of life that, while costly, is still desirable for parents as well as children. Also, could some of this money be better spent on other health problems, such as treating cancer, heart disease, or other chronic disease?

Much of the controversy deals with infants born at twenty-two or twenty-three weeks of gestation. A recent report out of the UK examined ethical issues raised by developments in medicine. The group, called the Nuffield Council on Bioethics, published guidelines saying that babies born before twenty-two weeks should not be given intensive care and should be allowed to die, while those born at twenty-five weeks should receive medical treatment to ensure survival.[17]

According to the Nuffield Council, babies born between twenty-three and twenty-four weeks can be given treatment if parents agree to it. But the prognosis of the babies help may color the decision of parents and healthcare providers as well as the situation of the parents. Is this a first child? Is this a last chance at pregnancy?[18]

Practices across the UK's roughly 250 premature baby units varies, but generally more are reluctant to resuscitate even at twenty-four weeks with survival rates hovering at 16 percent to 20 percent for babies born at twenty-three weeks, according to studies done in Norway and in the UK.[19] In the US, the reality is that even the American Academy of Pediatrics has a cut-off as to where medical intervention makes sense for preemies.[20] It seems that most doctors are on board with this notion. It is recommended to not resuscitate babies born before twenty-three weeks, while babies born

---

15. Behrman and Butler, *Preterm Birth*, 329–31, 399, 416 Table 12-8, 426 Table 12-9, 419–20, 420–21 Table 12-10; March of Dimes et al., *Born Too Soon*, 17 Table 2.1.

16. March of Dimes et al., *Born Too Soon*, 17 Table 2.1.

17. Nuffield Council on Bioethics, *Critical Care Decisions*, 156, par. 9.16e (note the recommended exception at 156–57, par. 9.19); also 154–55, par. 9.15; and 155–56, par. 9.16b.

18. Ibid., 155–56, para. 9.16.c–d.

19. Laurance, "The Big Question," paras. 5–6; also Costleloe, "Short Term Outcomes," 2012, e7976.

20. Aziz, "NRP Current Issues," 5–7, ; also Perlman, Jeffrey M., et al., "Special Report—Neonatal Resuscitation," e1329–30.

after twenty-six weeks are usually resuscitated. Survival generally improves with each passing week, but that is unlikely to give any additional reassurances to parents going through each passing day of hope tainted with uncertainty for what the future holds.[21]

My mother tearfully recalls all those years ago a hospital chaplain asking whether she wanted to baptize me before I was taken to the premature infant station. Unable to know for sure of my chances, she could only have hope that I was older than what I appeared, because of the lines on my hands and feet. Her choice had to be horribly guilt-ridden. A choice that was on top of a traumatic day that began with giving birth and not hearing me cry in the delivery room. Any woman who has given birth can tell you that your baby's first cry is the one that fills you with awe and immediate love for the little human that just took their first breath in this world. As I was my mother's third child, she immediately knew things were different when the room fell silent. And she already had had mounting apprehension that followed her being rushed to the hospital in labor nine weeks ahead of schedule.

They gave my mom the news of my size, and she eagerly and fearfully wanted to see me.

The urge of not wanting to touch or connect with an infant born far too early is something I'm sure many parents may have felt. And I wouldn't hold it against my own parents for perhaps feeling that way. Doctors also naturally react by not being very hopeful for the infant. At the same time it is hard to fight the urge to hold and love a baby that may not look anything like the healthy apple-cheeked Gerber Baby.

Consequently it is no wonder that doctors' views of resuscitation differ widely from those of the parents. Parents do not have a weight or age or conditional cut-off of any sort, according to academic studies. Conversely, doctors who know what may lie ahead for the child (disabilities, blindness, surgeries), may see the situation very differently—technological breakthroughs aside! According to a 2001 study from McMaster University in Ontario, a majority of people interviewed believed that all attempts to save premature infants should be made, while only 6 percent of health professionals said the same.[22] Studies in the US, according to pediatrician Dr. Rahul Parikh, come to the same conclusion.[23] Neonatologists William

---

21. Rahikh, "In Preemies, Better Care."
22. Streiner, et al., "Attitudes of Parents."
23. Ibid., Abstract; Parikh, "In Preemies, Better Care."

Meadow and John Lantos say that it used to be viewed that cerebral palsy was "God's fault," while now roughly half of cases are the fault of doctors, an issue they find "hard to live with."[24]

One story is that of Barb Farlow, who is now an advocate for patients and families.[25] She begins her story with receiving a diagnosis at twenty-two weeks pregnant that her daughter had a genetic disorder called trisomy 13 and 18—a condition commonly screened for in mothers aged thirty-five or older in the US. With this chromosomal condition, many babies die either before birth, during labor, or shortly thereafter. Only a small percentage survives beyond one year.

After being born full-term at 7-plus pounds and normal APGAR scores (a delivery-room assessment of a newborn's condition) of 8 and 9, baby Annie was able to come home after six weeks at the hospital. Annie's later complications at home required hospitalization when she was seventy-seven days old for suspected pneumonia; she was also considered for surgical correction of a narrow trachea, known as tracheal stenosis.

Whisked away to the intensive care unit, Annie wore a mask to help her breathe. A doctor asked Barb and her husband Tim if they should resuscitate Annie if she was to stop breathing. They said yes, as they understood their daughter to be suffering from pneumonia—a treatable illness. Later that night while coming to terms with the idea of Annie needing surgery for a narrow trachea, Barb and Tim took turns sitting with her. At one point Annie's vitals began to plummet. But there were no alarms and no nurses were present. The baby's primary physician arrived on the scene and told Barb and Tim that it wasn't pneumonia and asked whether they wanted to intubate Annie. The distraught parents decided that the surgery wasn't in their daughter's best interest and neither was life support. Annie passed away soon thereafter. It was only after going through medical records Barb and Tim discovered that a do-not-resuscitate order had been placed before they had provided their consent.

"I think the main messages that I would like to share really relate not only to children with disabilities, but to any vulnerable patient where the evidence-based statistics suggest that they will die soon," says Barb Farlow of Patients for Patient Safety Canada in a YouTube video.[26] "To try to

---

24. Meadow and Lantos, "Moral Reflections," 595–97.

25. For the following on Annie Farlow: Patient Safety Canada, "Circumstances of Baby's Death."

26. https://www.youtube.com/watch?v=XliZGuhHqx4.

see that through the parents' or the families' eyes or the patient if they are able and to understand what they understand and think about the condition, what their expectations are, and to respond to those expectations appropriately."[27]

After working with Dr. Annie Janvier, a Montreal neonatologist, and Dr. Wilfond, a Seattle neonatologist, Farlow had her story and those of others published in a paper published in the journal *Pediatrics*.[28] The paper challenged traditional views held about the challenge of raising medically fragile children, finding that the parents and siblings were happy in sharing their lives with disabled children. Dealing with the disabilities was nothing for the families as compared to the families' efforts to find doctors who understood what the parents were going through.

If those findings weren't enough to give doctors pause about basing a child's chances on statistics, Dr. Janvier has published numerous papers in neonatology and has worked with patients and families confronted with difficult decisions about withdrawing therapy, end-of-life issues, and decision-making in the face of uncertainty. Besides her work in the University of Montreal the pediatrics department, she holds a PhD in bioethics and is a clinical ethicist. She has examined why neonates are devalued compared to other patients, the personhood concept, and the subjectivity of the "best interest" principal in clinical ethics.[29]

Some of her most intriguing research looks at how the goals of fertility specialists often conflict with those of neonatologists. "To assume that extreme prematurity is the main ethical problem in neonatology, however is to jump to premature conclusions," she writes.[30] The large majority of preterm infants are between thirty-two and thirty-six weeks gestation and these "late preterm" births are what pose the largest emotional and financial burdens on families and society, she argues.

Focusing on the rising number of premature births, which she says are a consequence of the lack of government investment in preventing preterm birth, her findings suggest that society, babies, and families continue to pay more every year: financially, physically, and emotionally for the avoidable burdens of prematurity. All issues close to her heart, following her own

27. Patient Safety Canada, "The Patient Narrative—Barb Farlow," at 5:54 and 9:41.

28. Janvier et al., "The Experience of Families."

29. Sainte-Justine University Hospital, "Annie Javier," January 1, 2014, under "Publications."

30. Javier, "Jumping to Premature Conclusions," 659.

child's birth at twenty-three weeks. Her baby girl was in the so-called "optional" category for life support.[31]

Those early days were not easy for her and at one point Dr. Janvier and her husband decided to withhold care to baby Violette. Dr. Janvier wrote that she hated being encouraged to participate in her daughter's care. She has said she believes the urge to not bond too strongly with a premature or sickly newborn may be a protective mechanism for parents. Today Violette is a healthy girl, but not every story has a happy ending, as Dr. Janvier, who is also involved with palliative care for fetuses and neonates, well knows.[32]

She uses the example of Patrick Bouvier Kennedy, son of the late President John F. Kennedy, as a prime example of how far the technology has come. In 1963, he was born at a gestational age of thirty-five weeks and died two days later. Now babies born at thirty-five weeks have mortality rates only slightly higher than those of full-term infants.[33]

All developed countries have reported rising rates of preterm births, with the US leading the pack with 12.5 percent of births in 2004 being preemies. Babies that are extremely preterm, with a gestation of fewer than twenty-eight weeks or a weight of less than 1,000 grams (also called extremely low-birth-weight babies), comprise 0.8 percent of all deliveries and about 10 percent of NICU admissions. Currently, infants weighing 1,000 grams or born at twenty-seven weeks' gestation have an approximately 90 percent chance of survival, with the majority having normal neurological development.[34]

The cases that spark particular attention occur prior to twenty-seven weeks and these births hold greater the risks of complications, mainly developmental delay, cerebral palsy, chronic pulmonary disease, learning disability, hyperactivity, and, much less frequently, deafness and blindness. Babies of less than twenty-six weeks gestation, as noted, form a minority of babies in the NICU. Of the survivors, about half are without disability at three years of age, and 25 percent have a major impairment such as cerebral palsy (10 percent), blindness (2–5 percent), deafness (2–5 percent), and developmental delay.[35]

---

31. Parikh, "In Preemies, Better Care," par. 13.
32. Ibid., 13.
33. Javier, "Jumping to Premature Conclusions," 659.
34. March of Dimes, "Born Too Soon and Too Small in Arizona," 1–2.
35. Behrman, Stith Butler, *Preterm Birth*, 346–97.

For bioethicists such as Dr. Janvier the questions are very urgent. When do you intervene medically? Should a medical intervention be stopped once it is started? Who should be responsible for these decisions and how? The issues arise quickly and require quick thinking that could lead to perhaps long-term situations that could lead to even more challenging decisions. One of the most profound questions regarding human life, Dr. Janvier writes, is: "which life with disability is worse than death?"[36]

The majority of preterm infants are born after thirty weeks gestational age, and this group also reports increased frequency of disabilities, such as cerebral palsy. In order to substantially decrease disability rates from late prematurity in the population and NICU costs, one would have to let patients of twenty-eight to thirty-six weeks gestation die, according to Dr. Janvier.[37]

Complicating these ethical issues is that 25 percent of preterm deliveries are medically induced because of risk to the fetus or mother. This often occurs in multiple pregnancies of twins, triplets, or more, and the delay in childbearing is a significant and potentially reducible portion of the prematurity rate. Artificial reproductive technologies bear much of the responsibility for these trends. In vitro fertilization (IVF) is one source of multiples, as 32 percent of multiple pregnancies are result of IVF. Fifty percent of twins and more than 90 percent of triplets are born preterm and wind up in the NICU.[38]

The average maternal age in the US is also on the rise and women over forty years of age have a greater chance of delivering preterm. Also, as women age they look to techniques such as IVF to increase their chance of conceiving. This decision to rely on expensive fertility treatments becomes easier as older women have greater financial resources to use such techniques.

Women often put off childbearing until their thirties or early forties in light of the costs of childcare, the lack of time off for maternity leave, and lack of additional financial resources early in their careers that are necessary for raising children. Younger women have a significantly lower risk of giving birth preterm. Dr. Janvier points out that infertility is a health problem that brings with it conflicts of interest when it comes to relying on artificial reproductive technologies. IVF and other technologies are not

---

36. Javier, "Jumping to Premature Conclusions," 660.
37. Ibid.
38. Ibid., 661-2.

paid for or regulated by the government, thus creating discriminatory access to fertility treatments due to the cost of services.[39]

The use of IVF is often successful and has led to an epidemic of multiple births that create perhaps a greater burden on families and society. The so-called "octomom" is one prime example. Nadya Suleman gave birth to octuplets in 2009 after already having six older children through the use of IVF.[40] The public controversy and dispute over the children's long-term care sparked a controversy over the use of artificial reproductive technologies and an investigation of the fertility specialist involved. Initially denying that she was on public assistance, she later admitted in 2012 that she was receiving public aid.

Less extreme examples of IVF's promise and peril occur every day. Roughly half of twins conceived using IVF are preterm, some extremely preterm. Desperation for success can catch couples in an extremely emotional state and more willing to even want to ensure twins by implanting more than one embryo. The process also means greater success in impregnating patients with fewer treatment cycles and thereby the success rate of a fertility clinic also improves.[41]

Dr. Janvier concludes that in a society where the patient pays for IVF, there is a perverse economic incentive for both patients and doctors to take greater chances, risking complications for both mothers and babies. She is an advocate of better public policy to decrease multiple births. Regulation and reimbursement of artificial reproductive technologies is perhaps a start. The sheer cost of IVF forces multiple-embryo transfer in order to insure greater success. In countries such as Sweden, Belgium, Finland, and Denmark, where reimbursement takes place, the percentage of multiple-embryo transfer, which often leads to multiple pregnancies, is lower. Dr. Janvier calculates that multiple gestations following IVF treatments results in 17 percent of NICU admissions.[42]

"Rising prematurity rates and the continued unchecked epidemic of multiple births are a sign of political and moral failure," Dr. Janvier writes.[43] Still, NICU admissions continue to rise and as a result NICUs have become

---

39. Ibid., 661–2.

40. Associated Press, "8 facts about 'Octomom.'" See also the news articles cited in Wikipedia, "Nadya Suleman," 3–4.

41. Ibid., 662.

42. Ibid.

43. Ibid., 664.

the economic engine that keeps children's hospitals running, according to ethicist John Lantos.[44] All signs point to serious societal conflicts of interest.

The decision is not so easy from the perspective of doctors or parents. In the UK, one study suggested that annual health and education costs for children born extremely premature are two-to-three times higher at age six than those born at full term. Ethicists say that doctors should be aware of the costs and even the costs of governmental support for a child's care, but should not let those considerations drive their decisions.

Being born in 1973—the year that it was decided that an abortion can be done up until viability, defining "viable" as being "potentially able to live outside the mother's womb, albeit with artificial aid," adding that viability "is usually placed at about seven months (28 weeks) but may occur earlier, even at 24 weeks"—I have often pondered when a human being becomes fully human in our eyes.[45] Today many parents—such as those I am personally familiar with—have ultrasound viewing parties, where proud parents can rent a room in the hospital or even host such a party at someone's home to show the first images of their unborn child. You can now view a computer-generated video of your ultrasound used by the OB/GYN to screen out any abnormalities.[46]

I remember seeing my sons on a computer screen in utero and seeing their feet and arms and head move for the first time. They certainly seemed fully human and more real after hearing their heart beat rapidly at around five months gestation or roughly twenty weeks. While hearing that heart beat during an ultrasound or during a fetal stress test can almost be as awe-filled as hearing that baby's cries after birth, it still begs the question of how we as a society view life. After numerous genetic tests and screenings that determined probability for Downs Syndrome and a host of other disorders, we have more knowledge of an unborn child's potential for ill-health than my parent's generation could have ever been conceived. But when I was born my mother was considered "mature" to be having a baby in her thirties, and her physicians determined that age was a factor in my early arrival.

Yes, I tended to be behind developmentally in my early years and was part of special programs put on by the March of Dimes to help speed along my development, specifically talking and walking. I am told I didn't walk until eighteen months and didn't really speak until I was nearly

---

44. Lantos, "Hooked On Neonatology," 238.
45. Roe v. Wade, 410 U.S. 113 (1973).
46. Davidson, "Ultrasound Parties."

two-years-old. When I started school, again I was behind in some areas. But I quickly caught up, although my eyesight was impaired and through the aid of thick glasses I was able to focus on the blackboard.

As I look at all the variables and statistics regarding premature birth over the last fifty years, it seems that an infant's gestational age, sex, weight, and mother's age could make all the difference as to the vibrancy of the life these babies could expect to experience. I've been fortunate in that I was born at a time when incubators were widely available, I was a girl, and I was gestationally mature enough to have my organs fully formed. Also my mother at age thirty was young enough to have good eggs but old enough to know how to patiently take care of a baby with special needs.

My mother was told by one elementary school teacher that she didn't have much hope for me and my academic potential. Thankfully that teacher was wrong, as many of us are in our own evidence-based assumptions. I loved school and learning, completed my elementary and high school studies on schedule, and was an honors student in college.

Does technology determine when our life begins and the quality of life we will have or does our humanity draw the line in the sand to say when a life-saving measure is acceptable?

Thankfully often what one sees of a person's body—its size, shape, gender, or abilities—are not indicators of the true potential of one's mind or skill. Is that determined in the womb? Before we are conceived? Perhaps it doesn't matter, as we learn to deal with the hand we are dealt, relying on faith, family, and maybe even futuristic technologies to push us along.

5

Discovering Our Culture's Script
A Manifesto about Our Cultural Views of Bodyselves

Ann Milliken Pederson

WE SIMULTANEOUSLY IDOLIZE THE human body and desecrate it. Americans export highly sexualized, exploited, objectified, and violent images of bodies throughout the world, dressed in the clothes of our consumerism. We know what sells. Magazines advertise how to reduce flabby muscles and how to make decadent desserts, all in the same issue. Young boys and girls receive mixed messages about being strong and healthy and yet they are seduced by the advertisements sexualizing every part of them. While our "parts" may tell the story, they do so in an un-wholly manner. We must rediscover the parts within our whole, the individual within the community.

We are incredibly complex bodyselves, attempting to figure out what that means for our self-identity. While celebrating diversity of our bodyselves we long for the familiarity of that which is same. Fear and anxiety drive the suspicion we have of one another. The need for more and more propels the engines of our workload, the vacations we take, and the relationships we have. But we are rarely satisfied. We are socially networked and yet lonely and in despair. Advertising and media reveal images that are only skin-deep, but yet we do everything we can to repair and enhance our aging skins. We are caught—betwixt and between the need to fit into our cultural norms and the reality that very few of us fit that icon of normal and beautiful.

As Christians, we confess that God has created us in God's image. As Christians, we affirm that we are creatures, made for living in loving relationships with God and creation. We find ourselves in a culture that does much to deny this. We are caught between the cultural images of ourselves that we have made and the image to which God has called us. The Christian doctrine of the *imago dei* is not always in sync with who we are and more often than not in conflict with our culture's image of what we should fashion ourselves to be. In whose image am I made, produced, sold, and fashioned? To respond to this, I must look into the mirrors of the culture that surround me: at ads in the media, the latest fashions at the mall, the body types of models and superstars, health care promotions, and in video games. The reflection that I see in the cultural mirror reveals that I'm not up to its standard: I'm too old, overweight, not up on the latest health food crazes, and don't exercise enough. We snap pictures of ourselves on our iPhones, follow the map of the human genome, Twitter our current status, or surf the World Wide Web. I find the cultural image of "selfie" reveals much about our current American iconography. The Urban Dictionary defines selfie as:

> A picture taken of yourself that is planned to be uploaded to Facebook, Myspace or any other sort of social networking website. You can usually see the person's arm holding out the camera in which case you can clearly tell that this person does not have any friends to take pictures of them so they resort to Myspace to find Internet friends and post pictures of themselves, taken by themselves. A selfie is usually accompanied by a kissy face or the individual looking in a direction that is not towards the camera.[1]

This about says it all.

Yet, we surround ourselves with the technologies that we need to fashion who we think we *should* be: pictures of perfection. I think of all the products on the market geared toward women my age who are "aging" and want to appear "ten years younger." Millions of dollars are spent on cosmetic surgeries to tuck and nip the folds of midlife. Supposedly, we are free to be whoever we want to be (as long as we have the money and social status), to have the right to pursue our happiness (yet this is difficult to distinguish from the pursuit of instant gratification), and to overcome our

---

1. Urban Dictionary, "Selfie," def. 1, written 2009.

limitations of being human. All of this, of course, must be possible within our market-driven, consumerist culture. It's no wonder that we hope for the Snow White image of our bodyselves (which of course is sexist and racist and also unattainable). In fact, most of us are like the Dwarfs: sleepy, grumpy, and dopey. We are flawed and "dwarfed" by our cultural ideals of beauty and perfection. In whose image are we made? In whose image are we created?

The answers to those questions reflect the values of our culture. It might be tempting to think of culture or the media or the advertising business as the reasons we are seduced by these glitzy images. And yet, culture is not an abstraction that we can point to, but it is a system of living relationships in which we are embedded and embodied. Simply by living in the United States, I embody in some way the multiple and mixed up values and ethos of our way of life. Our journey through our cultural landscapes will tell us much about who we are as bodyselves: diverse and yet the same, parts and whole, subjects and objects. Our interpretations of who we are and want to be are as multifaceted and complex as we are bodyselves. While we have sought simple and comfortable answers to the complex questions about human identity, we will find none. Instead, we will explore a few images that I hope reflect the multifarious nature of what it means to be a human bodyself. The images are not comprehensive. They are simply snapshots of a much bigger human album.

We live in a techno-culture. We are techno-selves relating to techno-others. Descartes' dictum, "I think, therefore I am," can now be translated into contemporary jargon, "iPad, therefore I am." Or "iPhone, therefore I am." It seems as if every other day there is another article in *The New York Times* informing me about how "wired" I am, and what that might mean for bodyself understanding. We are in the process of becoming, but what are we becoming? Am I a cyborg? An android? Am I simply an extension of the gadgets that are tethered to my body? Is our projected personhood defined more by our Facebook status than face-to-face encounters? I can look into the mirror some days and wonder who and what I'm becoming. I spend more time wired to gadgets than in contact with "real" people. And even the distinction between "real" and "artificial/cyber" doesn't make much sense when I think about my bodyself.

Simply looking at how we use technology will give us hints about the shape of our bodyself. Maybe I've spent too much time reading science fiction novels like *Prey* by Michael Crichton (2003), or maybe it's that I'm fifty-six years old, but I'm in both awe of and fear about where technologies are taking me. My coauthor, Philip Hefner, asks us to look at our self-image when we gaze into the cultural techno-mirror. Whose reflection do we see? What kinds of bodyselves are we becoming? "Does technology tell us what we want to do, our desires for accomplishing things? Or does it tell us who we are and what we wish to be?"[2] These questions provoke us to reflect not only on who we are but who we will become in the future. Four images of the techno-mirror reflect our techno-culture and ensuing self-image:

> The techno-mirror shows us that we want tools to do things for us, and it shows us what we want done.
> The techno-mirror shows us that we are finite, frail and mortal.
> We see in the techno-mirror that we create technology in order to bring alternative worlds into being, worlds that differ from the actual ones in which we live.
> Finally, we see in the mirror that although we are busy creating new realities, we do not know why we create or according to what values—so we have to discover the reasons and the values.[3]

So, who do I find when I look into the techno-mirror of our culture? Sometimes the image I see is my bodyself wired to multiple connections, trying to do multiple things, in multiple settings. I am a kind of techno-hydra, tethered to gadgets. No symbols can more adequately portray our human condition than the icons we find on computers.

Icons are graphic symbols on a computer screen that represent an object or a function. More than seven or eight years ago no one had heard of Facebook, represented by a small icon, an "f" encased in a blue square. Now more than five hundred million of us are "friends" on this vast and fast social network started by Mark Zuckerberg. Facebook represents our new way of creating and sustaining relationships. I can be friends with people at my leisure, and chat instantly. Or I can ignore their requests to be my friend, and hide their annoying posts. The story of how Facebook was created is told in the movie, *The Social Network*.[4] I waited to watch it. I wasn't sure I really wanted to see it because I wasn't excited to see what it might reveal about not only who Mark Zuckerberg is but also who I am as one who participates in this vast network of "friends." The movie captured me with its rapid-fire dialogue and snapshots of a younger generation creating

2. Hefner, *Technology and Human Becoming*, 28.
3. Ibid., 34–40.
4. *The Social Network* (2011).

its own image. I was both mesmerized and repelled by Jesse Eisenberg's portrayal of Zuckerberg. Not dissimilar to what happens on Facebook with "friends," moments of genuine intimacy between friends did not happen and reality is a blurred vision of cyber, artificial, and wired connections.

The reviews that I read about *The Social Network* were even more fascinating to me than the movie itself. They are a cultural commentary. In *The New York Times:* "It's a resonant contemporary story about the new power elite and an older, familiar narrative of ambition, except instead of discovering his authentic self, Mark builds a database, turning his life—and ours—into zeroes and ones, which is what makes it also a story about the human soul."[5] Throughout the movie Zuckerberg remains the heartless protagonist who sucks everyone into his virtual web. The movie captures the sexism, rampant ambition, revenge, and power that typify much of American culture. Are we really turning into faceless, soul-less characters who only know how to "friend" someone who remains in the void of cyberspace? Or have we created networks of relationships that keep us connected in new and unimagined ways? The movie doesn't answer those questions; that's why it is so powerful. We are creating our own answers. Not everyone is a fan of Facebook. Critics abound. The gadgets have become extensions of our bodyselves. They are changing how we relate with one another by rewiring our brains. We can be so-called friends with someone across the planet, create revolutions through the Internet, and change our profile with a mere update. Adults are not the only ones who are addicted to their gadgets.

One of my favorite articles from *The New York Times* talks about how the latest toy craze amongst the younger set is not a stuffed animal or a pacifier. The latest and favorite toy for toddlers is the iPhone or iPad. Parents describe how they can appease their noisy children simply by giving them the iPhone. The toddlers become as hooked on the gadget as their parents. "It's a phenomenon that is attracting the attention and concern of some childhood development specialists."[6] When I'm driving down the street and pass the proverbial van, I can see the video screens playing movies to pass the time and to keep the children from annoying their parents. What we are passing on to the children that learn to communicate without much face-to-face contact? Not everyone is so excited about the toddler addiction to gadgets. Research shows that children learn best through active

---

5. Dargis, "Millions of Friends," 1.
6. Stout, "Toddler's Favorite," 1.

engagement that helps them adapt to the particular situation at hand. And interacting with the screen doesn't qualify as face-to-face contact. By the time they are teenagers and heading off to college, parents and children are enmeshed in the need to call each other and text dozens of times a day. No longer does the parent drop off and leave their child in the new and foreign world of college. While parents might remain empty nesters in one reality, they are fully engaged and hooked in with their children at another level. Now colleges are worried about the demands of parents who expect that their children text them several times a day and share their recent Facebook status updates.

I have been amazed that at the age of fifty-six I can find myself spending hours during the day lost on the World Wide Web. Pretty soon I forget where I am and I'm lost in the reality of cyberspace. After checking the updates on my Facebook account, rifling through hundreds of emails, I can still find time to scan *The New York Times* headlines and read other articles on different websites. What I have gained from such use of the Internet is quick access to lots of information, some of which is very helpful and interesting. However, I've also found that my students need help discerning how to use this information. Just because it's on the Internet doesn't make its content *true*, or even *real*. I've been able to keep in touch with friends that I haven't seen for several years. We share photos, anecdotes from our life, and occasionally write some interesting messages to each other. However, what I've also gained is an acute case of tendinitis. I've had to give up playing the piano and flute, and it hurts to type on the computer. I swallow anti-inflammatories every day, ice my elbow and hands and hope that someday the pain will go away. I could cut back on the time I spend on the Internet, but it wouldn't be easy. I am wired. And, I'm tired. I get tired of checking my work email, my home email, voicemail at work, voicemail at home, voicemail on my mobile. What I've gained through virtual reality I'm losing in other and maybe more important ways—peace and quiet. It's no wonder that along with our gadgets and technologies that we also long for places to disengage from all the chaos that they bring to our lives. I am embarrassed to realize that an evening can pass and my husband and I have spent more time with our faces buried in our phones than in the conversations we could have face to face. We are trying, with a modicum of success, to reengage by disengaging from our gadgets. We sit down in our living room to have a British version of teatime or sherry hour, and try to relax, having no agenda but just to share the small talk of the day.

Face-to-face interaction is how we learn. In early years when robots were being constructed, scientists and engineers used computer software programs and the "robot" looked like a detached mind in cyberspace. Descartes' dictum was embodied in digital flesh. But that Cartesian paradigm of embodiment is changing. What the researchers at the Massachusetts Institute of Technology Media Lab and Artificial Intelligence Lab have "discovered" is that, like humans, robots learn through social interaction. And not just any interaction, but it is through embodied social interaction. So, the new robots are made with human-like bodies—they are made to interact and learn with and through social connections. Just check out the homepage of Kismet, a robot created at MIT. The website notes: "Traditionally, autonomous robots are designed to operate as independently and remotely as possible from humans, often performing tasks in hazardous and hostile environments. However, a new range of application domains (domestic, entertainment, healthcare, etc.) are driving the development of robots that can interact and cooperate with people, and play a part in their daily lives."[7] Watch the videos of Kismet as it learns, literally, by interacting with humans. While some people might be fearful of what Kismet can do, for me it is a reminder of what it means to be a human bodyself. "Kismet is inspired by infant social development, psychology, ethology, and evolution, this work integrates theories and concepts from these diverse viewpoints to enable Kismet to enter into natural and intuitive social interaction with a human caregiver and to learn from them, reminiscent of parent-infant exchanges."[8] While much of our culture seeks to communicate in ways that are disembodied and antisocial, we are relearning, ironically, with and from our own created technological beings that we are social, embodied, and need face-to-face contact. What will happen to our bodyselves over the next decades as these social media technologies change and mold us? I don't know. Mostly, I am excited to find out, but not at the expense of forgetting that we are bodyselves whose most important way of learning about this world is through our physical, fleshly, face-to-face encounters.

Other technologies blur the inner and outer views we have of ourselves. Nowhere is this more apparent than from the views of how we reproduce. When I drive along the highways through the Midwest I can't help but notice the ubiquitous signs that usually have a fetus and an antiabortion message. Some of the signs will remark that abortion stops a beating heart,

---

7. Kismet Project, "Overview," first paragraph.
8. Ibid.

or that abortion kills children. On rare occasion the sign might mention the mother; however, that is usually in a negative manner, as if to say that the mothers alone are responsible for "killing" their children. However, what I find intriguing is that many of the pictures show only the fetus/baby and more often than not the baby seems to be floating in outer space, maybe tethered to something that might be the mother. In *Origins: How the Nine Months before Birth Shape the Rest of Our Lives,* Annie Murphy Paul notices that when the pictures of an embryo and fetus appeared in the 1965 *Life* magazine that as the photographer Lennart Nilsson "brought the fetus out of the shadows, he made the pregnant woman disappear."[9] Paul rightly notes that the fetus takes priority as an individual and its connection to the mother dissolves, as if the fetus were floating like an astronaut in outer space. Every detail of the fetus was clear, down to the nails on the hands and feet. "But for all their scrupulous verisimilitude, these photographs are missing the essential fact about a fetus, the preconditions of its existence: its connection to a pregnant woman. Without her in the picture, these images are no more than an optical illusion."[10] The body of fetus and mother become detached from what "really" happens in the nine months of pregnancy and fetal development.

Ultrasound has completely changed the way we view our bodies, even more dramatically for women who are pregnant. Annie Paul explains that originally "quickening" was defined when a woman first felt the baby kicking and moving within her. But now technology has changed this definition. She explains how at her own doctor's appointment the ultrasound changed her relationship to her baby. And this fascination can also turn to fear when we see what is inside of us by looking at what's going on outside of us. From x-rays to MRI, from PET scans to ultrasounds, science and technology take images of our insides and we see them displayed on the screens and printouts that our doctors hand to us or display in front of us. They are fascinating, sometimes in a Frankenstein sort of way. But like Annie Paul, when we can feel those images of our insides are not attached to a real body, to our body, then they can seem like illusions of what is happening. Inside and outside don't make as much sense anymore. They blur in our experience.

While it might seem like a leap from the fetus to the television, I can't help but recall a similar feeling of seeing images detached from the lives to

---

9. Paul, *Origins*, 123; Rosenfeld, "Drama of Life," 54–65.
10. Paul, *Origins*, 123.

which they are connected and how I become a spectator along the way. I see others "out there" in a separate electronic reality and they literally seem like objects upon which I gaze. I become a spectator of bodyselves, not a participant with others as a bodyself. When I travel to conferences or to do research, I will stay in the hotel and often late at night will turn on familiar news channels to see what has happened during the day. Conferences are especially strange because I can spend hours and often days sealed in rooms that separate the attendees from the rest of the world. And so to find out how the world "out there" is getting along, I attend to the news. While in Chicago, a city in which I once lived, I might hear about the local political scandal or updates on the Chicago Bears. If I listen to CNN or BBC, I hear and watch details about other people's lives in countries and situations far different than my own. And yet that is what is so strange. I am let into the horrific stories about victims of war, or the affair that some politician has had, or the scandal of an athlete's life. Like the fetus on the ultrasound or on the roadside sign, I can't really see what is going on in the bigger picture. The stories seem strangely detached from my conference-weary body that is curled up on the king-size bed in a generic American hotel, while I play an hour of Angry Birds on my iPad. We both long for intimate and loving relationships and yet more and more we merely connect online.

Face-to-face interaction will never replace the connections we have via social networks. And that is what we have—connections—through Facebook, Twitter, Instagram, and texting. But do we have relationships? I'm not sure that connections are the same as relationships. In an age where we wage war by sending un-"manned" drones to target the enemy, we lose the faces of those who suffer from the devastation. When we only connect, and never really relate, can we really expect our notions of community to give us anything but being "alone together."[11] I am hopeful that the college students that I teach are leading us in new directions. I met with a young woman named Dannika Nash who wrote something on her blog about what it means to be church. Without intending to have it do so, the blog went viral. Our local newspaper even did a story on her blog in which she wrote a challenge from her generation to the church. After I read her blog and visited with her at school, I wrote this as a response to her:

> To the young reformers in this new generation of college students:

---

11. Turkle, *Alone Together*, 2011.

To all the young people like Dannika Nash, a junior theology and English major at the University of Sioux Falls, I want to give thanks for your bravery and honesty. If trends reported in a blog by Martin Marty (church historian) are accurate, the confidence in religious institutions is on a decline. I'm not surprised by this fact, and it's not just people like Dannika Nash and those in her generation that are frustrated and disillusioned with the church. I can relate to much of what she is saying. Instead of giving up on the church, she is extending a challenge to the church to open its arms wide enough to embrace all those who it has tended to exclude. In her recent blog, she writes: (I invite you to read the whole blog): "But my generation, the generation that can smell bullshit, especially holy bullshit, from a mile away, will not stick around to see the church fight gay marriage against our better judgment. It's my generation who is overwhelmingly supporting marriage equality, and Church, as a young person and as a theologian, it is not in your best interest to give them that ultimatum."[12]

As I teach first year students about Martin Luther, I realize that her challenge to today's church is very similar to the confrontations that Luther had with the Papacy (language included). I invited her to come to two of my classes at Augustana College and speak about her theological views and her frustrations and hopes for the church. She ended one class session with the statement that topics like same-sex marriage are not just issues, but are about real people who matter. And the best way to encounter people is face-to-face. This statement, for me, defines incarnation: we meet God in the face-to-face encounters with those whom we love and those we consider enemy. And that's the hardest challenge I can think of in an era where we tend to de-face those whom we consider "other." We meet God in the faces of each other. While Twitter and the Internet, brought me to Dannika's work, it was the face-to-face conversation with this marvelous young woman and my thoughtful students that will give me hope about what it means to be church. I wonder if we can't find new ways to expand what it means to be church—yes, it is for Lutherans, where the Word is preached and the sacraments given. But today, I experienced flesh becoming Word, in the face-to-face conversations about what God's grace means in a world that is so defined by hate.

Joseph Sittler, a Lutheran theologian, challenged Christians to listen to the artists, poets, architects, scientists, and musicians to discover the

---

12. Pederson, "Ongoing Reformation," pars. 1 and 2.

pulse of the world, to hear and see what they bring forth about the nature of what it means to be human.[13] The church needs to hear that again. Maybe the words of Macklemore and Ryan Lewis in "Same Love" or the artwork by Marc Chagall also bring us Word.[14] God's love is expressed in the incarnational grace notes where we least expect them to be. And today, that was in a religion classroom with students talking about what church means to them. I am hopeful that connections are becoming relationships and that the church can be part of creating new communities that challenge the cultural view that *mere* connections are enough.

Looking back, I can tell that I am a child of the fifties and sixties because I still remember the scenes on the television set where the Marlboro Man herded cattle, and rode his horse into the sunset. What is it about this cowboy on a horse that conveyed such a powerful image of masculinity? On the frontiers of our culture, the "self-made man" developed its Hollywood bodyself in the likes of the made-up Marlboro Man and the true-grit of John Wayne. The Marlboro Man symbolizes American values of autonomy and progress—the expansion of the West. Mythic characters rise from advertising campaigns and none were known better than the Marlboro Man, the mythic cowboy of the West. Originally Marlboro cigarettes were advertised in the 1920s as a lighter alternative to regular cigarettes. In the 1950s, when health concerns related to cigarettes and cancer started to surface, companies started offering filtered cigarettes. Marlboro did not have one so they started to advertise a new filtered cigarette, but did not want it to be seen as a "feminine" way to smoke. They wanted to appeal to men, so using the advertising company of Leo Burnett they created the infamous Marlboro Man to sell this new cigarette.[15] By the 1960s this cowboy galloped across many a television screen. Ironically, three of the famous Marlboro men died of lung cancer.[16] Writer James Twitchell stated, "The Marlboro Man was strong, powerful. He never speaks. He's so tough. The genius of the ad is that at the same time there was a rising realisation that this thing will kill you, it was identified with a character who was, on the

---

13 Sittler, "Education as Furniture," 102–4.

14. Lambert, Haggerty, and Lewis, "Same Love."

15. Burnett, "The Marlboro Story," 42; also Marchese, "A Rough Ride"; Schalch, "Present at the Creation."

16. Schalch, "Present at the Creation"; and Pearce, "At Least Four Marlboro Men Have Died of Smoking-Related Diseases."

face of it, indomitable."[17] But Madison Avenue made the Marlboro Man become the epitome of what it meant to be a "real man." The Marlboro man joined the glitz of Madison Avenue to convey an American myth about a do-it-yourself culture where limits can be overcome.

The Marlboro Man is now a figure of a distant past, and we have replaced him with other cultural icons. Just think of all the thrillers or mystery novels where the main character (male or female) is a kind of do-it-yourself hero. In a series of nineteen novels (with more on the way) written by Lee Child between 1997 and 2014, the main character, Jack Reacher, epitomizes the autonomous man of American culture.[18] Reacher, an ex-military policeman, is mobile; he is free to be on the go where life leads him next. Almost like a modern day Robin Hood, or a "A [modern] Goliath who has a noble bent and an itchy trigger finger," he defeats the bad guys and helps those in distress, all with a great deal of violence.[19] Nothing ties him down and he is beholden to no one. Both men and women like to escape with Jack Reacher into a world that is not of their own making—where they feel trapped by their commitments. Mobility = autonomy in our culture.

To be a real "man" is to be free, to do what one wants to do. The American frontier was built on the notion that limitations can be overcome, that pulling oneself up by the bootstraps always worked. Politicians wage war with one another about how much we can expect the government to do for others instead of what we should be able to do for ourselves. We expect our bodies to overcome their human limitations. Illness is always cured, death is conquered, and nothing is far from our grasp if we have enough true grit and determination to make it happen. We don't really want to face death, illness, and our frailties. Of course, the irony is that the Marlboro man now symbolizes the cancer that overtakes our lungs, that costs healthcare industries millions of dollars each year, and sends thousands of people prematurely to their graves. We let our bodies be sold to Madison Avenue for the price of the smoke that rises into thin air. Ironically, the price we ultimately pay is denial of who we are created to be and what our bodies are for.

One of the first dolls that I was given to play with was the Barbie doll. I took extremely good care of her, not wanting to mess her perfect looking

---

17. Connolly, "Six Ads That Changed the Way You Think," par. 11 under "Marlboro Man."

18. For a list of Child's novels complete through 2014, see Child, "Lee Child Bibliography"; for more information about the outlook Child presents in his novels, see Curtis, "Curious Case."

19. Curtis, "Curious Case," par. 35.

body, and to this day I still have Barbie (and Ken, Midge, Skipper, and Skooter) in boxes stored in my basement. As a child, I don't know that I ever really thought about the kind of figure that Barbie had. But she became the image of what it meant to be an American woman. Barbie was the cultural icon of thinness when I grew up in the 1950s and 1960s. And while today the American Girl Doll might offer an alternative to Barbie, my fear is that young girls (and boys) are still surrounded with toys that play into pernicious visions of perfection.

Even more harmful models of thinness than Barbie are sneaking into the media, advertising, and Facebook ads luring young teenagers and women into obsession with their weight and figure. Everywhere women look they are encouraged to lose weight. Women and men are shaped by this Myth of Thinness: "Typically, the desire to lose weight begins slowly and subtly in responses to self-consciousness about our bodies."[20] We are bombarded with health-food ads, with the latest pill that will help us to lose weight, and with the killer exercise routine that will slim our bodies into the image we want. We are a nation that overeats; we suffer heart disease and diabetes in highly disproportionate numbers from the rest of the world. Men and women suffer alike.

Underlying this desire for thinness is the shame men and women experience about their bodies. When they look into their mirror, they see imperfections and flaws. We don't live up to the "ideal." Imperfection and the ideal are just two sides of the same shame. Most women think they would be much happier if they would just lose weight. Male athletes swallow steroids in order to build more competitive bodies. Is this "merely" a cosmetic desire? As religion professor Michelle Lelwica notes, "As long as you remain unhappy with your body, someone stands to profit. Your discontent is an exploitable resource."[21] Like the Marlboro Man, Madison Avenue cultivates the worship of thinness and the exploitation of our bodies. But who exactly is "Madison Avenue?" We are.

Some women are redefining what it means to be bodyselves. While there is much to find troubling about these new voices, I also find hope. In the 1980s, Madonna offended almost everyone with her renditions about how to be a material girl.[22] Her outlandish theatrics, however, empowered and changed the ways that women were part of the music industry. Women

---

20. Lelwica, *Religion of Thinness*, 63.
21. Ibid., 64.
22. Madonna, "Material Girl."

began to express their sexuality and gender identity for their own sake and not for the sake of pleasing men or Madison Avenue. And now P!nk (hereafter Pink) and Lady Gaga are doing the same, singing their new gospel about self-acceptance and empowering the underdogs. Their message reaches out to those in our culture whose bodies have been left on the margins of the mainstream. For example, when I listen to Pink belt out her ballad, "Raise Your Glass," I hear a message of grace about bodies.[23] The lyrics (and the images in the video) raise up those who have been downtrodden. From the underdogs and nitty gritty dirty little freaks, to all of us who have been enslaved to standards of perfection that we cannot meet, we listen to her words of liberation and encouragement. *The New York Times* recently reported that "Raise your Glass" was becoming the new ballad for those our society considers the outcasts, the underdogs—particularly young people who are gay, lesbian, transsexual, and transgender. These words of Pink offer hope to the downtrodden. I raise my glass to her.

What about Lady Gaga? I rather love her music and yet I also find her both repulsive and fascinating. In a recent post on Facebook, a writer talked about the theological implications of Lady Gaga's new song, "Born this Way." He writes:

> One of the song's concluding lines is, "Whether life's disabilities left you outcast, bullied, or teased, rejoice and love yourself today." This encourages separation of self-perception from the judgments of family, religion, and society. If you're different, it's the inability of the world to embrace or interact creatively, and not judgmentally, with you that's the problem—not the fact that you have listened to the call of your own truest self. The Church would do well to heed Sister's advice: Love people as they are, and "don't be a drag."[24]

You sing it, Sister Gaga. After hatching from an egg at the Grammies, Gaga reappeared later, draped by a black hat, covering much of her face, but also revealing the odd, fleshly protuberances that she had attached to her shoulder. Lady Gaga belts out a soteriological fashion statement about self-acceptance and love of the other.

In sports, the Super Bowl is a kind of religious event for American culture.[25] We participate in all kinds of rituals. Food is prepared and shared,

---

23. P!nk, *Greatest Hits— so Far!!!*, track 17; Meyers, "Raise Your Glass."
24. Parke, "Gaga Does God's Work," 2011.
25. Serazio "Just-How-Much-is-Sports," 2013; Wellman, "Super Bowl Civil Religion," 2014; Balmer "Tonight America Worships, 2014; Gardella, "Super Bowl Ads," 2014;

team clothing is donned, and chants are sung and yelled. I grew up watching football with my dad. As the only child, and female, my dad hoped that I would share his love for football. And I do enjoy the game. However, I'm also aware that Americans' obsession with football reveals the misogyny of our culture. Watching the commercials during the Super Bowl reveal as much about who we are as bodyselves as the actual game.[26] Much of the advertising in recent years has portrayed women as "chicks" or as showpieces for the men who appear as aggressive, beer-drinking hulks.[27] However, what really horrified me were the reports I heard about the side industry that has grown with the culture of the Super Bowl. Sex trafficking is now a feature of this annual event, and it grosses millions of dollars. *Newsweek* and *Time* reported that children are traded as prostitutes and men buy them for thousands of dollars.[28] Anti-trafficking groups collaborated to try and stop the sex industry. Katie Pedigo, an activist in Dallas, Texas, who wages war against trafficking, commented that about "15,000 prostitutes will be brought into North Texas for this year's Super Bowl."[29] "Approximately 10 percent, some 1500 women and girls brought in from out of town, will be abandoned here, left to fend for themselves once the festivities have ended."[30] Women and young children are bought and sold and then dumped. These horrific events are not confined to events like the Super Bowl; they are everyday occurrences.

According to a report from ABC News about sexual trafficking, Portland, Oregon, has the largest sex trade per capita in the United States.[31] Everything that is going on in Portland is happening in Sioux Falls, South Dakota and across the globe. Human trafficking commodifies and objectifies bodies. While this may seem like something that happens only in rare situations, the trafficking is a symptom of a culture that treats bodyselves like objects to be sold. I have been told horrific stories about young girls and boys in South Dakota who are the victims of trafficking. Whether during hunting season or the Sturgis Bike Rally, South Dakota's highways are arteries for trafficking. Federal agents monitor Internet sites like Facebook, Craigslist, and backpage.com for trafficking activity. Recruiters walk the

---

26. Burke, "For Some Fans"; and Bell and Aslan, *Ritual*, 153–54.
27. Covert, "Super Bowl Ads."
28. Goldberg, "Super Bowl".
29. Quoted in Sakmari and Stinchfield, "Pimps and Prostitutes."
30. Ibid.
31. Alfonsi and Fahy, "In Search of Love."

mall, come to college campuses, show up at truck stops and downtown areas.[32] As Susan Omanson, director of Be Free, a South Dakota organization to stop trafficking, suggested, the victims of trafficking need new "roadmaps" for their lives so they can begin to recover from the abuses and trauma of being trafficked.[33] Many of the victims are underage, from other countries, and from the American Indian reservations. Girls and boys are recruited as young as twelve and thirteen years old.

This modern day tale of slavery exposes manifold problems in our culture. In whose image are we made? If not God's, then whose? Who are our idols in whose image we remake ourselves? Maybe we can move beyond the imperfections of our mortal, finite, frail human bodies that we see in the techno-mirror. Maybe we can be trans-human or post-human. Maybe we just want to "improve" our bodyselves instead of perfecting them. Or maybe we merely want to fix the parts that don't work. But questions remain: How do we know what the boundaries are? What are the categories or standards for making those decisions? Who benefits from these options of improvement and/or enhancement?

Let's take sexuality as an example of how those who don't fit the cultural norm are asked to repair what separates "them" from the "us." In the United States, we assume that we are either/or: male or female. For example, how do we fill out an application for a driver's license: are you male or female? We check one or the other. And yet, for one in every one thousand births, the answer would be "both." There is no box to check. The science and classification of gender and sex fit the categories of our culture, but not the reality of those who embody it. Even the science of sex and gender selection is at odds with itself. And while slices of brains are studied for male and female differences, babies are born in hospitals where doctors and nurses have decided on the sex of the ambiguous, the intersex child not knowing what happened until years later. Why are we so uncomfortable with three or even five sexes, instead of two? Why isn't "both" an option on the driver's license? Do our pure ideas of sex and gender resist ambiguity?

These young bodies of intersex children, once relegated to freak shows or the circus, challenge our pure notions of male and female, of masculine and feminine. Do they need to repair their anatomy to fit the cultural standards? We are hearing from young intersex children that are now adults that they were disfigured and traumatized when they were forced at an

32. Don Jorgenson, "Dirty Little Secret."
33. www.befree58.org

early age to decide what sex they would be. And their parents often suffered with them, having no idea what to do in this oddly ambiguous situation. If what we are used to is a strict dualistic sex and gender classification of male or female, what on earth do we do with these little bodies? For many, their sex and gender are surgically chosen within a few weeks of birth. The child undergoes multiple surgeries, many of which can cause disfiguration and pain. What if the cultural gender status quo could change so that we accept more than two sexes? What if the sciences of sex and gender realize that our cultural view of gender doesn't cohere with reality and isn't natural for everybody?

Most Americans now know about Oscar Pistorius, who was "born without fibulas and had both legs amputated below the knee when he was 11 months old."[34] He ran with prosthetic devices in the last Olympics. In 2008, the International Association of Athletics Federation (IAAF) discussed whether or not he could compete in the Olympics. Questions were raised: "is it ethically right to enhance our species with the aid of technology or genetic interventions?"[35] This is hardly a disembodied issue and even though Pistorius ran in the last Olympics the issues have not disappeared. Pistorius's dilemma raises all kinds of questions, even those about the purity of the sport. Elio Locatetti, who is with the IAAF, questioned whether or not the purity of the sport would disappear. What on earth does "purity" mean? To be free of disabled athletes? He writes: "His case is a snap-shot into the future of sport. It is plausible to think that in 50 years, or maybe less, the 'natural,' able-bodied athletes will just appear anachronistic. As our concept of what is 'natural' depends on what we are used to, and evolves with our society and culture, so does our concept of 'purity' of sport, and our concept of how an Olympic athlete should look."[36] What appears as natural will soon seem anachronistic. How we define "normal" has to do with our cultural status quo and the evolution of ideas in our culture. And so this experience of the culturally normative body is rooted in our techno-cultured bodies.

The most recent book that has captured my imagination, in both good and frightening ways, is called *Generosity,* written by Richard Powers (2009). Set in Chicago, a failing author is hired to teach a group of students at a small arts college in downtown Chicago. He gets to know one

34. Camponesi,. "Oscar Pistorius, 639.
35. Ibid.
36. Ibid.

of the students and becomes alarmed by how happy she is all the time. She comes from Algiers and has experienced life-threatening, nightmarish trauma. After speaking with the college therapist, they decide together to find out what makes her this way. She eventually becomes a specimen for those to examine under the microscope of psychologists, trans-humanists, and genomic engineers. A British transhumanist (thinly disguised as a version of Aubrey de Grey, a theoretician in the field of gerontology) becomes involved and wants to research her DNA with the hope of engineering people's moods.[37] Many of us hope to surpass the limitations of our body and the swings of our emotions and moods. If only we could be enhanced. If only we could change. If only we could be happy all the time. But the novel conveys the price that will be paid if this happens. In a sense she is reduced to just her DNA—she becomes a body of information for others to examine. We are hardly condemning the kinds of technological, medical, and scientific enhancements that genuinely enhance the quality of our lives. But when we seek to improve the human condition, we must simultaneously be aware of what we mean by the "human condition." For Christians, that has something to do with being created in the image of God. And that means we are endowed with the freedom and responsibility of being created co-creators with God. Who we are is what we become through our relationships with each other and with God. That says a lot about being human.

---

37. SENS Research Foundation, "Aubrey de Grey," par. 2.

6

Where Medicine and Christianity Collide

Ann Milliken Pederson

IN LIGHT OF MEDICAL science and biotechnologies, what does it mean to be a human person? In light of the biblical narrative and Christian tradition(s), what does it mean to be a human person? For most Christians, those questions don't come together into the same focus unless they experience a crisis or life-changing event regarding their health. In exploring both questions, the convergence of what is happening in medical science and biotechnologies and in the readings of the Christian tradition will reveal that we are amazing, complex bodyselves who are called to be creatures of God, alongside the rest of creation.

The human condition defies simplistic explanations. Nowhere is this more apparent than in the practice and science of medicine: they reveal that bodyselves are mysterious and messy. We often talk about medicine and healthcare as if they are ideas apart from the people who practice them. Medicine and healthcare are not about abstract thoughts; they are practices done by specific individuals and groups of people. In other words, medicine and the delivery of healthcare are cultural practices; they embody the ambiguous values of our culture toward bodies. We simultaneously promote the health of the whole, but sell the parts, protect the rights of individuals, but forget the community from which they came, improve and enhance some bodies while simultaneously dispensing with and ignoring others.

All the relationships that we have that connect us through space, time, and with others make us who we are. These webs of relationships began before our birth and extend through a lifetime to our death. One observation that seems obvious: those relationships are changing at an exponentially fast pace. Most of the time we are unaware what is happening. In the arena of medicine and biotechnology, the pace of these changes is faster than our reflection on them. Ethical issues seem to arise almost every day in ways that we couldn't have imagined a week or two before.

In his provocative book, *The Creative Destruction of Medicine,* Eric Topol claims that humans have become *homo digitus:* species in which digital technologies extend and entangle the meaning of what it means to be human. The book describes "both how the creative destruction of medicine can and will be achieved and how we will arrive at a knowledge of individuals so fine-grained that we can speak of a science of individuality."[1] Topol's vision is that the digitization of medicine and of how we relate together will converge to create better medical care—more individualized, less expensive, and more hopeful for curing diseases that incapacitate us. While many people like myself have feared that digitization will overcome individuality and create a cyborgian collective nightmare, Topol offers the opposite, a dream that responds to the needs of each person and that each person will "be seen and treated with utter respect for his or her individuality."[2]

Topol criticizes medicine and healthcare for being too focused on the "mass market" and not on the individual. Medicine and healthcare (and the biotechnology associated with them) are in a crisis. His solution: "We need real evidence based on individuals, not populations. Fortunately, our ability to get just that information is rapidly emerging; beginning an era characterized by the right drug, the right dose, and the right screen for the right patients, with the right doctor, at the right cost. Medicine for the common good is not good enough. Now let us see how to get something better."[3] Topol's critique of medicine raises the longstanding problem of our modern worldview: the dualistic understandings that we have of ourselves and of our relationships to the world around us.

---

1. Topol, *Creative Destruction of Medicine,* 228.
2. Ibid.
3. Ibid., 32.

Much of the contemporary worldview of self and other, body and spirit emerges from our epistemological ancestry. "I think, therefore I am" becomes a caricature of who we think we are: body parts that need to be fixed or improved, a mind that is separate from our body, a spirit that will leave our body when we die, a body that is untouched by the trauma of finitude and mortality, bodies that are instrumentally helpful to the work of our "true self," which seems trapped in a vessel, and finally we see ourselves as superior and set apart from the rest of creation and creatures. Coupled with these views is a certain paternalistic elitism that renders doctors above and apart from the patients. But this is changing with a speed that neither patient nor physician can seem to grasp. Topol writes: "Up until now the medical community has been the privileged, nearly exclusive source, purveyor, and reservoir of all health and medical information. The Internet and the unprecedented growth of online, health-oriented, peer-to-peer networking, however, have forced a rapidly approaching parity of knowledge between the public and the medical profession."[4]

Healthcare, technology, and medical knowledge have come to a great "convergence" according to Topol that will revolutionize how medicine is delivered. At the end of his book, he writes: "Now we are ready to discuss the implications of this series of convergences and perhaps the greatest convergence in our history: the one that finally coalesces the rapidly maturing digital, nonmedical world of mobile devices, cloud computing, and social networking with the emerging digital medical world of genomics, biosensors, and advancing imaging."[5] We have become *homo digitus*. We are not a new species, but a species that is constantly becoming something new and complicated, entangled and extended into webs of relationships that become more complex every day.

Topol claims that medicine can become more individualized, treating each person respectfully through the complex webs in which they are embedded. Our individuality emerges through networks. In a similar manner, we revealed in the previous chapter that we are embedded in and emergent from our evolutionary past. To quote a famous African proverb: "I am because, you (plural) are." This shift in an epistemological aphorism will help us unravel what it means to be human amidst this new convergence of knowledge and technologies. As always, the result is ambiguous.

4. Ibid., 227
5. Ibid.

On the one hand, as consumers of healthcare we believe that if something can be done to improve our lives there is a moral obligation to do it. We expect physicians to use various technological means to intervene, prevent, enhance, cure, and overcome our limitations. We also reduce our bodies to parts that can be fixed, sold, and exchanged. For example, eggs and sperm can be sold legally in much of the United States, while kidneys cannot. The dominant culture sets the standards of perfection, while those in the minority are forced to assimilate. Veterans whose limbs have been shattered by the tragedy of war can find artificial substitutes with prostheses and therapy. The elderly whose joints have been worn down by age can have hip and knee replacements. The neonatal intensive care unit (NICU) keeps premature babies alive who otherwise would have died. Targeted genetic therapies personalize treatments for people with cancer.

Medicine is a double-edged sword; it provides the care and extension of life for many and yet it also fails large populations of peoples who cannot afford the care. Whether through direct interactions with those in healthcare and medicine or through its unavailability and absence for others, everyone is shaped by the stories that medical science and biotechnology tell. The stories, however, are not simple, as Phil Hefner reminds us:

Living in Paradox
i am vibrant
embodied personality
motion enfleshed
unpredictability on the move

yet here
i submit myself to
empirical fact
impersonal and predictable

living flows matched
to charted norms
pulsing organs caught
in frozen images

technoscientific
practice is not me
cannot capture life

yet self depends on
lifeless knowledge

more techno
enters so deeply
attaches so firmly
i am technoself
cyborg is who I am

while who I am
still observes
a twoness
contesting with
the oneness

always
a someone
in itself
more than flesh
more than tech
and knowledge

is this soul
or wishful dream
or actual
paradox

TECHNO-BODYSELVES

When I think of what it means to be a bodyself in light of medical science and biotechnologies, I'm transported into what seems like another world—that of science fiction. The speed at which new technologies are changing the life I have known as familiar are moving faster than the light we can shed on the impacts of these changes. I grew up watching *Star Trek* and *Star Trek: Next Generation*. Spock was the ultimate embodiment of the rational, logical side of human life. He remained detached and objective at the most critical times. He was half Vulcan, half human—a hybrid of sorts, a chimera of the human self. Commander Data arrives with the crew of the next generation—an android whose goal was to become more human. At some point, an emotion chip was embedded in Data. Like Spock, he was the most intelligent of the crew, whose intelligence was created artificially. In an episode entitled, "The Measure of a Man," Data is legally declared to be an autonomous individual like all the other humans on board the Starship Enterprise. He is no longer considered property of the ship. Data became almost human. The main characters of these great science fiction epics of the twentieth century are androids, Borg, and hybrids. Who are we? We are cyborgs of co-created flesh and machine, nature and culture, biology and artifice. From the hours we spend on the Internet, to the androids we carry in our pockets, or the machines to which we are tethered for life support, the boundary in our bodyselves between machine and human, artificial and natural, is difficult to distinguish. We are hybrids, chimeras of the opposites we try so hard to keep apart.

Technology is most integral to and connected inside of us when we are born and when we die. I'm a fifty-six-year-old married woman with no children. I'm not sure why I'm interested in the sciences and technologies of reproduction, but I am entranced by what I am learning. Questions I have include: What point in embryonic development does personhood start? How do the various forms of contraception interfere with the reproductive process in embryonic development? What are the causes of infertility? What does one do with unused and unwanted embryos? Does the embryo have rights? What are the rights and responsibilities of a parent? What are the different types of stem cells? Should a couple have a second child as a source of stem cells for a first child with a disease? What will we find out about pre-implantation selection and elimination of genetically defective embryos? What further manipulations of the genome will be possible? I cannot comprehend all the ramifications of what is happening in the sciences of reproduction and development. But what I do know is that we cannot stop asking the questions, seeking answers, and being open to being both critical and appreciative of what the sciences are illuminating about the bodyself.

Recently, I had two experiences in one day that jarred my worldview: one was while I attended grand rounds at our local hospital, the other while I drank my morning tea and read an article in our local newspaper about Native American children. The experiences butted up against each other, revealing the extremes of what it means to be born into this world. I went to the OB/GYN grand rounds about pre-implantation genetic screening and diagnosis with a colleague and friend, Dr. Maureen Diggins. During part of the presentation, we watched the video of one cell being extracted from an eight-cell embryo. Dr. Diggins leaned over to me and said, "Isn't that the most amazing thing you've ever seen?" Dr. Diggins' amazement and wonder at the human body is contagious. I would even venture to say her scientific research becomes a religious experience for her—she gains insight into God's creation.

Later on that same day when we had attended grand rounds, Dr. Diggins and I talked about the article in the paper that we had read, about how South Dakota has the highest infant mortality rate in the United States. We agreed that somehow medicine and technology must also assist those who want to have children but whose hopes are dashed in different ways. For Indian children surviving birth is an onerous job. The white media often stereotypes Indian mothers, blaming them for problems because they drink too much. But this simply isn't the case.[6] Most people don't realize that mothers in the tribal communities in South Dakota consume no more alcohol than other people in the state.[7] The reservations are geographically large, far from urban medical facilities, and transportation is not always available, so many mothers cannot get what they need in order to have adequate prenatal care or for taking care of their child after the delivery. The journey from mother's womb to the world is complicated, even dangerous. And the journey remains complicated after the child is born in their world where poverty and violence create nearly impossible odds for success.

Technology has reshaped when we are born and how we survive the first few days and months. Because the possibilities of having children through artificial reproduction technologies has increased so greatly, children come into the world prematurely and their lives are saved and extended through the resources of the neonatal intensive care unit (NICU). In a gripping book, *The Lazarus Case: Life-and-Death Issues in Neonatal Intensive Care*, John Lantos takes the reader through the ethical, medical, and existential tales of the NICU. Lantos's narrative reads more like twisted, interlocking knots than a straightforward plot. He begins by describing three pillars in the landscape of Chicago where the stories are set: "The Sears Tower, temple of retailing, rising like a soaring bar graph above all the rest; the Amoco Building, built on energy, oil, and the antitrust laws that

---

6. Young, *Surviving Birth*.
7. Ibid.

broke up the Rockefeller oil monopoly into competing cartels; and the John Hancock Building—insurance—a monument to our efforts to escape the tyranny of chance."[8] The story about a premature baby in the NICU is told from the perspectives of the parents, physicians, nurses, and other family and caregivers. Nothing is simple and the technology complicates the plot.

Decades ago, as Lantos notes, the incubator was a technological wonder. The incubators were financially lucrative for hospitals and soon everyone felt morally compelled to use them. The same has happened with the NICU. The American dream of progress, of improving the human person, grows alongside the economic means by which it happens. In the NICU, tiny babies seem like cyborgs—hybrids of machine and human.

Lantos writes:

> There is probably no eerier place in a hospital than the NICU. One enters thinking that one is prepared to see tiny babies. But the babies are unimaginably tiny. They are magical. They look something like the strange *Life* magazine pictures of babies inside the womb. The babies seem almost, but not quite, human, almost, but not quite, fetal. In their chimerical, half-human, half-machine state they seem not only helpless and pitiful but also exotic, threatening, futuristic, feral, untamed, barbarous. They evoke a strange mixture of sympathy and disgust. Their vulnerability calls out to us, and we want to help them, but there is also something repulsively bug like about them that makes us want to obliterate them. They shouldn't be there, so vulnerable and so dependent on the machinery and technology of medicine.[9]

Lantos captures what so many people feel and think when they have been in a NICU. We are techno-flesh, born into a world tethered to multiple machines. And many of us will leave life the same way.

Fourteen years ago I was diagnosed with uterine fibroids. During the last years, I was hospitalized twice for severe anemia. And then I had myomectomy surgery to remove a large fibroid on the inside of the uterine wall. During that procedure, a vein was nicked, my blood pressure dropped, and I was seriously ill. My husband and mother recall the tense hours while they sat in the family waiting room where every hour or so they would receive a call that updated them on what was going wrong. The surgery was supposed to last ninety minutes and I was to be back at work in about

---

8. Lantos, *The Lazarus Case*, 1.
9. Ibid., 28.

forty-eight hours. However, the surgery lasted almost six hours. I spent six days in the hospital, had a 10-inch incision, and took six weeks off of work to recover. And to make matters worse, I continued to have problems with bleeding from fibroids located outside the uterine wall, and the hormones used to treat everything caused high blood pressure over the years. Finally, a couple of years ago a different doctor suggested robotic surgery for a hysterectomy. This time the surgery lasted a couple of hours. I was in for a twenty-two hour stay in the hospital, had three small incisions (about 1–2 centimeters) and spent less than a week in recovery. The process was amazing and I have been very grateful for the technology of the daVinci Surgical System, and for my very skilled and compassionate surgeon.

When I was wheeled into the room for surgery I was asked if I wanted a glimpse of the da Vinci robot. The nurse told me that my surgeon would be seated at a large, ergonomically correct terminal with "four interactive robotic arms, a high-performance vision system and patented EndoWrist instruments."[10] The actual camera is about the size of a pencil and it takes three-dimensional images during the surgery. Sanford Hospital's motto of "improving the human condition" came true for me. I can only imagine what the future will hold for surgeons as more technologies are created to offer less invasive options for the patients. Robotic surgery can improve the outcomes of both open and laparoscopic surgeries. The daVinci Surgical System is composed of three parts: a console for the surgeon, an inside vision system, and a surgical cart, all of which give more control to the surgeon. The Surgical Cart and EndoWrist Instruments include "a camera arm, 3 working arms, a mobile base, and robotic parts."[11] The FDA cleared the use of the da Vinci Surgical System for the use in OB/GYN surgeries in 2005, and future innovations are now planned in robotics. The speed at which the technologies move can barely keep up with the surgeon's ability to train on them. And of course, for the patient, like me, I was happy to have a briefer time in the hospital and to return to work sooner than if I had open surgery. I am grateful to be techno-flesh, an embodiment of technology and body.

Indeed, the worlds of science and life-enhancing technologies are not fiction and they are here. Our future has arrived and we must ask what difference does it make to our self-understanding and to our future as a species? Some people think that the sacred is separate and unrelated to these

10. Davincisurgery.com, "Features," par. 2.
11. Ibid.

worlds of medicine and technology. But I claim that God is not apart from our embodied techno-selves, but indeed is in, with, and under these relationships with technologies and medicine. Where is God in the middle of all this? Precisely in the midst of these relationships that we can be assured that God promises to be present for us in the healing and transforming procedures that are part of the world of medical science.

"MINDING" THE EXTENDED BODYSELF

I attended a conference in September 20–23, 2012, at Akademie Loccum, Germany, sponsored by the International Society of Science and Religion on the theme of embodiment and embodied cognition. While I admit that I knew nothing about the field of cognitive science, I went to the conference hoping to learn more about the philosophy and psychology of mind. What I learned there not only affirmed much of my earlier theological and philosophical convictions, but also opened up a wider field of vision for how I interpret how we "mind" the world around us. I think of the famous London posters from the underground: "mind the gap." Every time I would step off the tube, that same voice would repeat the familiar words: "Mind the gap." The gap in my world was the one between mind and body, and now I'm learning to "mind" the world in wholly new ways.

Those who are in the field of embodied cognition explain that the way we see and know the world is inextricably connected to how we interact with the world. This feature of embodied cognition is called extended mind. "In this view, the mind leaks out into the world, and cognitive activity is distributed across individuals and situations. This is not your grandmother's metaphysics of mind; this is a brave new world."[12] This challenges the Cartesian notion that our minds are inside our bodies. While this understanding of extended mind remains controversial, at both scientific and philosophical levels, it has at least provoked me to think that the way we see the world is embodied, situated, and interactive. These embodied interactions might be more than just a cause and effect relationship with mind, but might indeed create cognition.

Extended cognition and embodied cognition draw upon the work of people like cognitive science philosophers Andy Clark, David Chalmers, and Alva Noe. Clark argues that the extended mind thesis is a better theory of cognition than the more "conservative" view of embodied/

12. Robbings and Aydede, "A Short Primer on Situated Cognition," 8.

situated cognition that says "certain cognitive processes lean heavily on environmental structures and scaffoldings, but do not hereby include those structures and scaffoldings themselves."[13] He explains that the temptation has been to locate all of cognition acts within the head and central nervous system. However, there are local operations of cognition that move between and amongst the brain, body, and world. "In this view, the mind leaks out into the world, and cognitive activity is distributed across individuals and situations."[14] As Clark explains, the "goings-on" are not bound to the brain or even the body. He labels his position the Hypothesis of Extended Cognition (HEC) and the more conservative position Hypothesis of Embedded Cognition (HEMC).[15] This hybrid nature of explaining cognition is similar in spirit to what Donna Haraway, a feminist philosopher of science, does with the collapse and implosion of traditional boundaries. She also claims that the pervasive dualisms of mind-body, culture-nature, nature-human implode into the web of relationships between the bodyselves and their environments.[16] These views of embodiment challenge the traditional Cartesian mind-body "problem" and have important implications for a theology of embodiment.

Often I hear people saying that our "true selves" are not our "outward selves," as if there is some inner chamber that is untouched by this vessel that houses the self. However, like it or not, we are our bodyselves. Those of us who have been steeped in the Western Enlightenment traditions have been trained to think that our minds and bodies are separate. Or from another point of view, some voices in science and philosophy claim that our minds are nothing but the neural connections in our brains. The new fields of embodied cognition challenge both these views. We construct our minds through the bodies with which we engage the world around us. Our knowledge is not only embodied, it's also situated. Cognitive psychologist Barbara Tversky writes: "The world serves not just our own minds but also our communications with other minds: a glance at the door tells a partner it is time to leave; the salt and pepper shakers on a dinner table act as props in a dramatic retelling; here, that, and this way can be understood

---

13. Clark, "Curing Cognitive Hiccups," 163.
14. Robbings, and Aydede, "A Short Primer on Cognition," 8.
15. Clark and Chalmers "The Extended Mind," 7–19.
16. For example, Haraway, *Modest Witness*.

efficiently but only in context."¹⁷ Or another way to put this is: "Cognition is not just situated, it is also embodied, in ways that are hard to untangle."¹⁸

After listening to and watching a TED talk on extended mind by David Chalmers, I was thinking about "where" in the world we are, if the where outside our skull is indeed part of our extended mind/self, then our location in the world is also extended as a bodyself. As an example, Chalmers explains how we feel we lose our memory when something like a fire or flood destroys family artifacts like pictures. We have off-loaded our memory into the stuff that we have lost in the tragedy. I can think of other situations where this link between extended mind and memory are related in ways I had not considered beforehand:

1. Loss of a partner or friend who is so intimate that they share our mind—when we finish someone's sentences. In grief, we speak and feel that nagging sadness that something of our self is gone.
2. When Jesus comes back from the dead and Thomas asks to see and touch Christ's wounds, a sense of loss is restored. Resurrection is more than some kind of spirit; it restores that painful sense of loss.
3. My iPhones and social networks are extensions of my mind/body self. These really change social interactions with those around me.
4. How I am testing students is changing. If students have the use of Google at their fingertips, it might be more important to teach them how to critically retrieve and interpret information than simply to memorize it.
5. Graveyards are extended memory banks of who we are.

How does the world reveal itself to us? Minds are located in an ecological environment. This translates into how we "take into the world," of how we "see the world." Seeing and interpreting the world are hermeneutical acts of the bodyself. Where we stand and where we interact literally determine how we interpret/see the world around us. The reason that we don't notice some things or perceive them is because we don't ask the right questions or come with the right background to notice them. Our background knowledge, even in our sensory motor skills, shapes the way we perceive the world. We make up our minds quickly, on the fly. The very ways we interact with the world shapes the way we see and understand the

---

17. Tversky, "Spatial Cognition: Embodied and Situated," 201.
18. Ibid., 202.

world. What is available to us comes from a place based on the skills and knowledge we bring to it. Seeing and thinking are interrelated hermeneutical processes.

What is the "mind's eye" or the link between perception and mind, seeing and knowing? We extend our mind into the whole environment. Clark's example that the notebook we use to put down directions to help us remember how to get somewhere is part of our "mind" and part of our knowing. If we extend the mind, we extend knowing to all. We can extend the "image of God" to more than just humankind. Not only do the sciences of embodied and situated cognition challenge this view, but so also do the sacramental and incarnational theologies counter this narrow view by claiming that God is not present somewhere "inside" of some spiritual chamber in our heart or head but instead that God dwells in all that we are and in all with whom we are in relationship.

We learn to think and communicate in, with, and under our body's relationship to the world around us—to paraphrase Luther. We get new knowledge in a sensory-bodily way that changes how we perceive the world. He claims that "our perceptual consciousness of the world as a causally, spatially, temporally well-ordered, regular, and predictable place depends on the world's actually being that way. . . . The world is not a construction of the brain, nor it is it a product of our own conscious efforts. It is there for us; we are here in it."[19] What we designate our "mind" extends into and is created with the interactions it has with its environment—from the body to those places, people, and events around the body. Perception, action, and thought create each other.[20] Noe asks, what is the domain of where consciousness arises? Consciousness is not something inside of us. It is an event, a process. Consciousness is less like digestion and more like dance: involves the environment, placement in a landscape, social connections, and our whole bodyselves. Consciousness does *not* happen from a "brain's eye" view alone. Contrary to the Cartesian view, we are not merely trapped in our brains as selves. We are already at home in the world. Where we are is after all who we are. The bodyself is an "environment" of relationships and consequently perceives and interprets the world within that environmental context. Perception is an activity as well as interpretation. "Perception is any activity of sensorimotor coupling *with the environment*."[21]

19. Noe, *Out of Our Heads*, 142.
20. Robbins and Aydede, "A Short Primer," 4.
21. Noe, *Out of Our Heads*, 80.

David Seidel, a college professor and philosopher, uses an example of how the arts can help us to literally and metaphorically see in new ways. "One of the most enjoyable aspects of teaching art history to college students is presenting to them an artist or work of art with which they have been long familiar, perhaps Michelangelo and his famous *Pietà* or Marcel Duchamp and his infamous *Fountain,* and opening it up to reveal something they hadn't noticed, taking it out of their familiar categories and re-enchanting it."[22]

For example, the first time that I saw Monet's *Haystacks* was at the Art Institute/Chicago. Instead of moving around in an oval, walking from one painting to the other, people stood in one place and turned their body around to look at the paintings. Simply the way we moved changed the perception and interpretation of the artwork.

We move from here to there: embodied and extended cognition teaches us that our bodyselves are where our "minds" begin and extend with and into the world. Seeing the world is thinking about the world, and with the world. Diana Eck, a scholar on world religions, talks about the hermeneutics of the visible in a way that is very similar to what the cognitive psychologists and philosophers are speaking about with embodied and extended cognition:

> Seeing, after all, is an imaginative, constructive activity, an activity of making. It is not simply the reception of images on the retina. The term *hermeneutics* has been used to describe the task of understanding and interpreting ideas and texts. In a similar way, we need to set for ourselves the task of developing a hermeneutic of the visible, addressing the problem of how we understand and interpret what we see, not only in the classical images and art forms created by the various religious traditions, but in the ordinary images of people's traditions, rites, and daily activities which are presented to us through the film-image.[23]

In a similar manner, art historian David Seidell writes the following about putting art and theology together:

> Theology has been the means by which I create that necessary space to allow art and culture to operate with its own integrity rather than as tools for politics or even virtue formation. My work has been committed to revealing art to be a cultural practice that

---

22. Siedell, "Haystacks and Shadow," par. 1, my emphasis.
23. Eck, *Darśan*, 14.

enables us to experience our humanity—our creatureliness—most deeply, and even where the tremor of a "deeper magic" of grace, which contradicts the forensic nature of the world, can be felt most powerfully.[24]

Both Seidell and Eck know that hermeneutics, or the art of interpreting the world around us, is an act of the whole bodyself in relationship to the world around it.

At a conference in Germany, a colleague challenged me to expand and extend my vision of what it means to be created in the image of God by reading not only the theologians from my Western/Latin tradition, but also the writings of theologians from the Eastern Orthodox traditions. Like the work of the cognitive psychologists, philosophers, and neuroscientists, the writings of the Eastern Fathers, particularly Maximos the Confessor, extend my Western reading of incarnation, the sacraments, and embodiment. Word and words, Logos and logoi, come together to open the incarnation of God to all things. A prominent thinker and author on religion and science, Christopher Knight, writes: "These logoi, through inhering in each created thing, are not themselves created. They are, for Maximos, nothing other than God's presence in each thing: a manifestation of the Logos itself."[25] Western theologians frequently focus the lens of the incarnation through Anselm's famous questions: why did God become human? This question is usually answered by an explanation that God comes in Jesus to save us from our sins, through his death on the cross.[26] However, theologians like Maximos the Confessor challenge this narrow reading with the notion that if humankind had never fallen God would still have become incarnate in the person of Jesus Christ, simply for the sake of God's love for humankind.[27] God's home is in this world, in us, just because God likes to hang out with us!

So, I can take this expanded vision of the incarnation and extend it to claim and include all of creation within the image of God. Knight suggested that Eastern Orthodox understandings of the incarnation might offer just this kind of theological support for a re-interpretation of the imago Dei. He writes: "For Maximos, this understanding led to an expansion of what Philip Sherrard has called the Greek patristic understanding of 'the universality

24. Siedell, "Theology & the Arts," par. 3.
25. Knight, *The God of Nature*, 98.
26. Ibid.
27. Ibid.

of the Incarnation,' in which the Logos is seen as incorporating itself 'not in the body of a single human being alone but in the totality of human nature, in mankind as a whole, in creation as a whole.'"[28] Incarnations and images of God are visions of the creation's relationship to its Creator. East might meet West in claiming that all of creation reflects both the incarnation and image of God. I know that my vision of the West must be met by a correction from the East.

MULTIPLE IDENTITIES IN MULTIPLE BODIES

What about those who have been left out or ignored by the "advances" of modern science and the benefits of healthcare? What are their stories? I know that I'm among the privileged in this world that have access to good healthcare and resources. So, I must listen to and ask about those people who are left out by those who are in power and who control the availability, quality, and access to healthcare. However, such inquiry is never without difficulties because dangers arise when those who are "in the conversation" try to speak for those who are "left out" of the conversation. To try and attend to these difficulties, I offer my concerns. First, I must always acknowledge, as much as I am able, my own standpoint and biases, while simultaneously being open to hearing from others about limitations of my perspective. Secondly, listening to and telling stories and asking about others' points of view, requires time and a willingness to learn new ideas. Thirdly, learning how to understand how things work and what might be possible, requires that I pay attention to other ways that stories become available: through media, the arts, popular culture, literature, and everyday conversations. I begin with the stories of all human bodyselves, but particularly with those whose lives have not mattered or have been forgotten. The way is not always clear; the roads are not always on the maps of those who have created them.

A year ago at Augustana College, I listened to a public lecture by Dr. Lionel Bordeaux, who is the President of Sinte Gleska University on the Rosebud Reservation. Bordeaux took us on a journey through his life from White River, South Dakota, to Black Hills State University where he received his undergraduate degree. He explained that South Dakota is failing Indians, not only in education, but also for healthcare and other basic needs. Those of us in the room were quiet as he explained that the Euro-American

28. Ibid.

systems don't honor the Lakota values of tribalism, respect for elders, compassion, and working by consensus. Around 80 to 90 percent of people on the reservation struggle with poverty and a disproportionate number are unemployed. The Rosebud Reservation has one of the highest suicide rates per capita in the world. Suicide rates for Indian youth are the highest in the nation and five to six times higher on reservations in the Northern Plains. Bordeaux claimed that the United States has a "fourth world" right in its borders—a world often plagued by illness, high suicide rates, extreme poverty, and depression. When the tribal nations were imprisoned by white civilization their freedom was taken and consequently their joy and love of life. He explained all of this without anger or blame to a white audience, most of whom were academics.

One way to kill somebody is to disembody them by taking away their customs, language, and culture. Any Native expressions of religion or social activity were banned. There were diverse Native peoples at the Hiawatha Asylum for Insane Indians who spoke different languages and came from different parts of the country. Many were shut away in rooms for decades and couldn't communicate with others. The Lakota people, whose wisdom was discounted and nearly lost, still struggle with reclaiming their rightful identity. In more recent years, members of the Lakota Nation's Yankton tribe hold religious ceremonies in honor of their friends and family members. The metaphors and myths of madness still resound in the halls of medical institutions in the early twenty-first century. We put away or drug those we deem "impure." Will those of us in the white culture learn our lesson? That depends on how willing we are to face what we have done in the past and to then change how we live in the future.

Pemina Yellow Bird explains that the situation symbolizes much of what is left out and ignored in the dominant narratives about medical science, technology, and health. The state of healthcare on the reservations reflects the tragedy that poverty and racism inflict. She writes: "We also fight to keep what is left of our homelands, cultures, languages, intellectual, cultural and property rights. Our loved ones are dying in unprecedented numbers from heart disease, diabetes, cancer, substance abuse, and sheer heart-sickness. We have the highest rate of suicides of all ages, we have the highest rate of infant mortality, and we have the lowest life expectancy of any group in the United States."[29] Despair and anger abound on reservations. Yellow Bird challenges Native peoples with what she calls three magic

---

29. Ibid., 3.

questions: "We must ask ourselves: (1) what happened to us? And, (2) these things that happened to us, how are they affecting us today? And finally, (3) we must look among our original teachings, values, and instructions to re-discover what we must do to take good care of ourselves."[30] She rightly explains that no one else can do the work. Families, tribes, and nations must express their despair and anger. It's a matter of life and death. Hope comes when stories are told and listened to with deep compassion. What is horrifying, of course, is that this is just one story among hundreds or even thousands. What follows is a more recent version of the horror story.

As a way for the white culture to control the number of American Indians being born, sterilizations of Native women occurred at rapid rates on the reservations during the 1960s and 1970s.[31] Women were not given adequate information for consent, and in many cases were sterilized against their will. In an article by Jane Lawrence, she reports: "Native Americans accused the Indian Health Service of sterilizing at least 25 percent of Native American women who were between the ages of fifteen and forty-four during the 1970s."[32] While the Indian Health Service improved healthcare conditions for Native American women, there were still egregious acts committed against them. The nature and lack of informed consent and the attitudes of the physicians that did the sterilizations were simply ignored at first. During the 1960s, sterilizations in large numbers were performed not only on American Indian women, but also on Hispanic American and African American women. Physicians thought they were helping the society at large by controlling the number of births in families who were poor. Hundreds of women were sterilized without their consent. I am sickened not only by what has happened in the past, but also, even more so, by what women continue to face today simply by living on a reservation and being poor. One in three women living on a reservation will be sexually assaulted. And sexual assault is one of the main reasons that Indian youth attempt and succeed at suicide. Over and over, bodyselves are judged for their worth and value by the "norm," by those who are in control and have power today. Native Americans have tried to resist assimilation into the dominant white culture. But like those caught in the power of the Borg in Star Trek, the web of power and domination is too much.

---

30. Ibid., 3.
31. Lawrence, "The Indian Health Service," 400.
32. Ibid.

The plot repeats itself. Nowhere else in the twenty-first century is this more apparent than for those who are gay, lesbian, bi-sexual, and trans-sexual/transgendered. I had a student a number of years ago who spoke to a group of medical residents about diversity and why it was important to remember that there are multiple ways of being a woman and of being feminine and masculine. She told them that she was lesbian and while she understood that physicians needed to ask her if she was pregnant before they did certain tests she became weary of explaining again and again to the same physician about why she wouldn't be pregnant. It was as if the physician couldn't comprehend that she wasn't sleeping around with men. Her story made me think again and again about the assumptions made about gender and sexuality.

The former student has now been ordained as a pastor in the ELCA, who recently voted to approve individuals for ordination who are GLBTQ and are living in committed relationships. *The Argus Leader,* our local paper, features Megan Rohrer in an article: "Rohrer, 30, is the first openly transgender Lutheran pastor ordained in the United States. Transgender is an umbrella term for people whose gender identity or gender expression differs from the sex they were assigned at birth. Only a very few choose to change their bodies through hormones or surgery."[33] Megan's grandmother who still lives in South Dakota has argued in support of the ELCA's decision with those who disagree about Megan's ordination. I have watched as my own church struggled to make a decision which would include the bodyselves of those they had previously considered to be unworthy to be ordained. My home synod in South Dakota voted against the ELCA's decision. Why was this story featured in the newspaper? It is not just news for the ecclesiologically minded. It is about our bodyselves—those who have been ignored and excluded, and those who do the ignoring and excluding. Megan's story shares many of the same dimensions as the one about the Hiawatha Asylum for Insane Indians. Both share our culture's inability to deal and face differences, with hybridity. To be face to face with one who is "other" is to face one's own fear. Our cultural expectations blind us from recognizing and being compassionate towards those who don't fit "our" standards of purity and perfection. The very language of "us" and "them," "ours" and "theirs" betrays the tragedy of the divisions created within our bodyselves and within our corporate bodyselves. I have a lot to learn.

---

33. Callison, "Transgender Minister," first par..

CANCER: ON BEING HUMAN AND COMPANION SPECIES

I can think of no other illness that affects more people in our culture in the early twenty-first century than cancer. In fact, the US government felt that cancer was such a threat to the wellbeing of its citizens that in 1972 it officially declared war on cancer. The story of cancer in twenty-first-century America is a complicated plot with multiple characters. Nearly everyone has either had cancer or knows someone who does. Cancer does not just affect individuals; it affects entire families and communities.

Almost three years ago my mother was diagnosed with breast cancer. She was eighty-five years old. Her mother died from breast cancer when she was seventy-eight. Her maternal aunt also died of breast cancer, and possibly her grandmother. And I have had two biopsies for suspicious findings on mammograms. Amazingly, however, since most of the women on the maternal side of my family were older when they were diagnosed with breast cancer, my chances of getting it are no greater than the normal population. That has not diminished my anxiety a great deal, however, when I get a mammogram. At some level, all women wonder and worry about that test that could reveal their one in eight chance of getting breast cancer. Lying face down on a table and being punctured with a large needle to extract cells from the suspicious site is an experience I do not care to repeat. The procedure itself was not nearly as painful as the couple of days that I waited to find out the results. The statistics for being diagnosed with cancer are much higher as we age. So, when my mother was diagnosed with breast cancer, we initially didn't worry too much about it. She was often told, "At your age, cancer grows very slowly, and you could die of something else, before the cancer kills you." We have grown to hate the phrase, "at your age." While dealing with breast cancer is different for someone who is eighty-five than someone who is thirty-five or even fifty-five, it is still an experience that led my mother and me, as her companion, into territories we had not anticipated. She crossed a threshold, with me as a companion, from health to illness.

When my mother received the final pathology report that her kind of breast cancer was HER-2 positive and estrogen receptive positive, we had virtually no idea what that meant. We learned that about 25 percent of breast cancers are HER-2 positive, and it can be one of the most aggressive forms of cancer, even for someone at "her age." My mother went from thinking that the lumpectomy was a procedure for taking care of "the lump," to a diagnosis that would send her into a year of receiving Herceptin treatments, thirty-five treatments of radiation, taking an estrogen blocker, and connecting with a world of oncologists, radiologists, and patients we didn't know existed.

The making of the drug called Herceptin, this powerful weapon in the arsenal against cancer, exemplifies how the story of the war against cancer unfolds. According to Mayo Clinic:

> HER2-positive breast cancer is a breast cancer that tests positive for a protein called human epidermal growth factor receptor 2 (HER2), which promotes the growth of cancer cells. In about 1 of every 5 breast cancers, the cancer cells make an excess of HER2 due to a gene mutation. This gene mutation and the elevated levels of HER2 that it causes can occur in many types of cancer—not only breast cancer. Trastuzumab, which specifically targets HER2, kills these cancer cells and decreases the risk of recurrence. Trastuzumab is often used with chemotherapy.[34]

The story of HER-2/Neu in breast cancer treatment is one that brings together those in medical science and biotechnological research into a fast-paced, action-packed thriller. In her introduction to Robert Bazell's *Her-2: The Making of Herceptin, a Revolutionary Treatment for Breast Cancer*, Dr. Mary-Claire King talks about this modern tale of science and technology: "This, then, is a fable for our time. It is one with many tragic losses and an ultimate happy ending, or at least one that is hopeful. It is a complex biological mystery; a drama of high finance; a series of non-sentimental, intelligent love stories; and a terrific vindication of stubbornness in a good cause. In all, it proves that good science makes a great yarn."[35] I had never imagined that I would be mesmerized while reading a detailed story about the creation of a treatment for breast cancer. That is until the breast cancer was my mother's.

We often act as if cancer is something that invades our bodies from the "outside." Yet, cancer comes from within us—from the very growth of cells that also create life as well as destroy life. This view of inner and outer creates deeply personal and intimate questions for the one who is ill. Robert Bazell writes: "Our bodies are metaphors of who we are in nature, including all that is "natural. . . . Cancer, the uncontrollable multiplication of cells, has existed the moment single-celled organisms joined together to form multi-celled plants and animals. . . . Growing and dividing is the most basic

---

34 Pruthi, "HER2-positive."
35. King, "Introduction," xiii.

function of individual cells. It is the impulse by which life has survived and evolved for billions of years. Every cell in our bodies carries this evolutionary force."[36] Some patients have a sense that their own body is destroying them, and ironically it feels personal—as if their cells were "ganging" up on them, a kind of medical guerilla warfare. Guilt often ensues. Patients will ask what did I do to deserve this? Family members will goad them about habits like smoking that might have caused the cancer.

On the one hand, if cancer is viewed as an "invader" from the outside, we use advanced weapons to target and destroy the invader. And for many patients, chemotherapy is the ultimate medical experience of these weapons. Unfortunately, as we spend billions on the "war against cancer," we often neglect the limitations of how much war our bodies can withstand. We try to overcome disease, conquering it with "magic bullets." There is a seduction to surgery—we can simply remove the diseased part and get on with our lives. Our bodies become images, anatomical charts, numbers, and parts. On the other hand, if cancer is something that comes from within us naturally, then we might figure out ways to treat cancer, not simply as an alien enemy to be destroyed, but as a part of who we are that needs to be listened to, observed, and figured out. How we see where cancer comes from may have an impact on the way we can heal from the illness (which is different than curing the disease). In *Speak the Language of Healing: Living with Breast Cancer without Going to War*, the authors challenge the traditional battle imagery of going to war against cancer, and consequently waging war on our bodies. The four women, all of whom had cancer and wrote about their experiences, do not surrender their hope for a cure or their desire to be healthy. What they do give up is the notion that cancer comes from some alien source, or that it was a punishment for something that they had done wrong. They understood what Robert Bazell did: that cancer is part of who we are. "Cancer was not an enemy to be vanquished, but a part of ourselves."[37] And they treated their bodies with compassion and acceptance instead of anger and frustration. Approximately one in eight women will be diagnosed with breast cancer, and it is the second leading cause of death for women. Women are not statistics in a war. Cancer is personal.

A couple of months after surgery, my mother began seven weeks of radiation. I often came with her to the oncology center and during the first week she was tattooed at the sites where she would receive radiation. Now,

36. Bazell, *Her-2*, 12.
37. Kuner et al., "*Speak the Language*," 10.

I listen to women tell their stories about receiving these strange "badges of courage" that helped to save their lives. But the marks never go away and are always there to remind them of the days of pin-point technologies that literally sear away the residual cancer cells. After the seven weeks were complete, she received a diploma and a card of congratulations from the man who attended the front desk at the cancer center. He always welcomed us every time we went and now when my mom returns for scans or blood work, we can count on his great smile and greeting.

That's part of the strange new world that we became inducted into during her treatments. From radiation, my mom became part of the infusion center, where every three weeks she received an infusion of Herceptin. Since she didn't receive chemotherapy, she didn't have a portable catheter (the portacath) surgically inserted and so the nurse would insert an IV. Since I have experienced the wonders of Picks and Sticks (the anesthesia specialists) because I don't have good veins for an IV, I always felt relieved when my mother's IV was inserted with seemingly great ease. Tylenol and Benadryl followed. As the year went on, two of my colleagues with whom I worked were diagnosed with cancer and began receiving chemotherapy. We would see them at the infusion center and my mom would be greeted with encouraging words and vice versa.

People shared their bodily experiences in ways that I could have never imagined. I remember one woman in the radiation waiting area showing us the burns she had experienced and how much hair she had lost. Others would sit silently, but look at my mother with eyes that were sympathetic. My mother never lost her hair, was never burned, and tolerated the Herceptin with very few side effects. I'm still amazed that after all the treatments, and now at eighty-eight years of age, she looks better than ever and is very healthy. Not too long ago she was told by her oncologist that she could come back in six months—a reprieve of the every three month blood work checks for the tumor marker. No doctor appointments, no blood work, no scans. At least for the time being, I am grateful. And I'm also grateful for the life of one little mouse who changed the course of cancer research.

A laboratory mouse that has been genetically modified, carrying a specific gene called an oncogene, is called OncoMouse. The gene makes her susceptible to breast cancer. OncoMouse is the first patented animal in the world. She is a metaphor of techno-science and techno-culture (and techno-humans). We buy, sell, experiment on, and patent animals. Of course, the story of the lab mouse is not so simple and neither is the self-understanding of the humans who created it. The story about OncoMouse emerges like the self-understanding of the disease of breast cancer—through complex interactions of technology and nature, machine, and humans.

The scenes from the stories of bio-technology and medical science are intimately connected to our cultural narratives. OncoMouse was created with the sole purpose to study and hopefully cure breast cancer. Such sacrifice we can applaud, but we must do so as we bear in mind the means to the end—to cure cancer. For the means to the end is not an innocent one. How we understand our relationship to OncoMouse tells us much about how we understand ourselves and our relationships with those around us. We have not always understood those relationships in ways that benefit all involved. Our practices require bearing witness to the consequences. There is no innocent storytelling.[38] What we are learning about our bodyselves and our "self-understanding" is that we are no longer simply and purely human, nor are the animals around us. The borders we once thought were closed between technology and nature, human and non-human are more open and fluid than we could have imagined. What began as an idealistic and optimistic cure for cancer has developed into a multi-billion dollar enterprise of research, economics, power, and politics. Stories about salvation, whether religious or scientific, share this ambiguous and messy legacy of culture.

Cancer reveals the pathologies of our culture. We know that race and economic status shape who and when someone gets cancer, who receives treatment, and how research monies are used. The privileges of race, class, and gender leave behind those who are not part of the "normal majority." Why do some people receive better treatment than others? To answer this question requires listening, reading, and researching in places and with people that are often neglected. We forget to think about whether transportation is available for people to get to the treatment, whether people have insurance, whether they can take time off from work to get to a doctor. Even meeting the expenses of recurring deductibles with people who have good health insurance can create extreme hardship. All healthcare facilities are not created equal. This is surely the case with cancer. A patient's history reveals a great deal, but it takes a nation of good diagnosticians and interpreters to change these alarming trends. Statistics are not just numbers; they reveal stories about women and men who suffer from the impoverished

---

38. Haraway, *When Species Meet*, 82.

way those who are ill are diagnosed and treated. Lots of voices still don't matter to the research and study of cancer.

I would love to think that cancer no longer holds the stigma it once did. But when I talk with those who have cancer and have lost their hair from chemotherapy they talk about how people stare at them in the grocery store. They know that the wig is not their real hair. Those who have cancer can still seem like the untouchables in our society. Friends and relatives are afraid to show affection to their loved one who is ill. No one knows what to say. Cancer is still a cultural stigma in many ways. And it affects every bodyself in this country, whether by having the disease or knowing someone who does.

BODIES AT THE END OF LIFE

All of us will age, get older, and die. It's the human condition. All the wrinkles, age-spots, sore joints, and gray hairs warn our bodies that they are wearing out. We sell multiple creams, laser surgeries, dyes, and ointments to counteract the effects of aging. For some, aging is not just part of the human condition that should be accepted, but it is a disease that, like cancer, must be fought and destroyed. Aubrey de Grey, a British engineer and scientist, along with others in groups like SENS, are using research to combat the diseases of aging.[39] He claims that our bodies are simply machines and if we can fix the parts (at the cellular level) we can usher in new immortal lifetimes for people. He hopes to rid our culture of the expense that fragility and aging causes. Through his scientific research, other benefits could come: a cure for cancer, for example. However, I worry that a culture that is already so obsessed with youth and perfection will find more reasons to ignore those who are vulnerable, frail, and alone.

However, many physicians who teach in medical schools challenge de Grey's notion that the human body is simply a machine. Like de Grey, they study the parts, but they also realize that the human person is much more and that this mystery of the more is what makes us human. Physicians learn not only the practice of medicine, but also its art. And the composition of the human body is the *magnum opus*. Daniel Callahan, one among many voices, challenges what he describes and labels as the "modernist" view of aging: (1) Medicine and biotechnology should wage a battle against aging like the "war against cancer"; (2) Humans can always bring about a better

39. SENS Research Foundation, "Executive Team," n.d.

future using science and rationalism; (3) Individuals are autonomous and should be offered the possibility of this life-extending science.[40] Underlying the modernist view, according to Callahan, is our fear of mortality and finitude, the "limits" of the human condition.

Callahan calls for a radically different view on aging than that of de Grey's. Using language that almost seems religious in nature, Callahan suggests that the elderly see their purpose in life (vocation) as service to the broader community, and especially to the young. Only the elderly have a perspective on time, and passing of the generations, that they can impart to the younger generations. The elderly can pass on the virtues of courage, humility, patience, benevolence, hilarity and vigor of spirit in face of their aging and pending death. We should emphasize intergenerational responsibilities instead of individual rights and personal choice. And we must talk publicly and openly about limits and boundaries of healthcare and the dangers of the sciences of life extension like those espoused by de Grey.

Another challenge to the views of de Grey and other transhumanists emerges from those who work in hospice and palliative medicine. Palliative care physicians explain that how we live is how we die. And we need to learn how to accept anMd face our death. Death does not necessarily need to be a medical defeat or create hopelessness and meaninglessness.

What is death? Christine Montross writes with such compassion and tenderness about dissecting cadavers that she breathes life into the subjects whose death she is learning from. When she first "meets" the cadaver, Montross ponders the "parts" she dissects: "The box bumps against my leg as I take it to my car. During the entire walk, I am thinking, this used to be a person in this box, and no one knows it." Although the cadaver is obviously dead, Montross learns as much about life and its mysteries. She reminds us that we really don't know as much as we think about dying and the definition of death. Life and death can still be a mystery to be explored and not merely a problem to be solved or cured. In a provocative statement, Montross says:

> Scientifically I side with the neurologists who designate death as the irreversible cessation of all functions of the entire brain. Philosophically I wade into murky and controversial matters with personal beliefs that the boundaries of death are nebulous. To me the definition of "dead" may extend far enough toward life to include a person whose brain is a physically functional void: the end-stage

---

40. Callahan, "Settzehants," 48.

Alzheimer's patient, for example, who never wakes but breathes and sends urine from injected liquid fluid into her diapers.[41]

The boundaries blur between life and death. Our life stories reveal the journeys of our bodyselves, told through the tales of medicine and healthcare. Our journey reveals that the road we have been on is neither straight nor narrow, but wide and full of detours, just waiting for us to discover the mysteries that lie ahead.

With this in mind, what have I learned about being a bodyself? About this blood and body that are given to me by God the Creator? A Christian perspective should welcome the advances of medicine and biotechnology that offer healing and hope to those whose lives are cut short by debilitating disease and suffering, should claim the reality that life and death are not in the ultimate control of humans, and can claim that it is precisely in human flesh that God works in the world. Our bodies are a mystery and our response to that mystery must be awe, wonder, and humility. The more we learn about our bodies from medical sciences the more humility we need about what we do with that knowledge. The human bodyself is a work in progress. What is happening in medical sciences and biotechnology is moving at such a fast pace that most of us don't know how to think through the implications of those changes. What it *means* to be a human bodyself is a work in progress, a process of translation and interpretation of massive quantities of information. We are technosapiens: bodyselves constructing our meaning about life in, with, and through technologies.

The categories and boundaries that once helped us understand who we are and what makes up our bodyselves no longer seem to work and that can be an opportunity for learning. We can only understand who we are as we place ourselves in others' stories, paying attention to the details. We are mortal and finite—that is part of being human. What we do with that seems to be up for grabs. One of the most important lessons I have learned from reading memoirs of those who have had cancer is that compassion and hospitality might be the most important lessons we can learn about what it means to be human. We extend hospitality when we welcome others into our lives. This is a powerful way of understanding what it means to not only be an individual bodyself, but to live in, with, and through each other. Finally, I believe that what it means to be created in the image of God is extended to all of creation. As humans, we are created co-companion species with those around us. And our relationships with other creatures

---

41. Montrose, "Body of Work," 34.

are complex and messy. Because we come from the *terra firma,* and God is the ground of our being, I define the image of God as: *the vocation of the created order to be and become freely that which fulfills God's gracious purposes and intentions for the creation.* Specifically, for human beings, I use the definition that my co-author, Philip Hefner, uses: humans are created co-creators, and the meaning and purpose of human life comes from their placement within the natural world. Are we "just another creature?" Is there something distinctive about being human? What does it mean to be a person? Do personhood and human qualify as the same definition? Can other creatures be non-human persons? Humans are bodyselves who have to live with the understanding that our relationship with the rest of creation is highly ambiguous and often very sinful. One of the challenges that I face as a Christian is to delve much deeper into how I live with, in, and under those around me.

7

A Scientific Take on Our Bodyselves
What Science Tells Us about
Our Bodies and Ourselves

Philip Hefner

EVOLUTIONARY SCIENCE ESTABLISHES—UNASSAILABLY—THAT SELF is body. In this chapter we explore how science makes this point and what it means for us. Some years ago, I had an experience that brought it home to me in an unforgettable way. A young man, who showed promise to become an exceptional pastor, arrived in his first call after graduation from seminary. At every step of his preparation, he had proved himself to be unusually well-suited for parish ministry—everyone expected great things from him. It was a shock when in the first months of this activity he was unexpectedly overwhelmed by a deep and disabling depression. He pulled the shades, turned on the TV, and stayed in bed. Weeks went by before he consented to a thorough medical and psychiatric assessment, as a result of which he went on a strict regimen of psychotropic drugs. Within an amazingly short time, he returned to his former self—for more than twenty years he has served vibrantly in his chosen calling as a pastor. To put it bluntly, this man was restored to a full life by a bottle of pills. Of course, things are not so simple, but the truth is that scientific knowledge, applied by technology to produce appropriate drugs, worked on his body—his brain—so as to affect a wholesome change in his mind, his emotions, and his behavior in ways that restored him to an energetic and satisfying life of effective service to others. That "bottle of pills" symbolizes a wide range of scientific research and knowledge that focuses on the body, with the aim of impacting our mind and spirit—our very selves, in other words. It also symbolizes that our bodies and selves are inseparable and interdependent. We are bodyselves. This story has been told many times in recent decades by people who have found themselves in the same situation as my friend—so frequently that although it is a dramatic event in people's lives, it is almost commonplace. Such stories are the background for saying that science shows us in unassailable terms that our selves are body.

Yet, most people put body and mind, body and soul, body and self in two separate worlds. A *New York Times* writer illustrated this chasm between body and self in a column entitled, "These Wretched Vessels"—that title refers to our bodies.[1] The writer's aim is to reject the notion that we are defined by the shape and condition of our bodies. So far, so good, but he goes on to speak of body in a way that excludes brain and mind—as if they are some kind of "spiritual" alternatives to body. "Our bodies are not ourselves," he writes:

> we can be dealt a set of imperfections—of crushingly severe limitations, in fact—and nonetheless transcend them, with some help and some luck and, above all, some grit. That we can look as far beyond the flesh that we've inherited as we resolve to. . . . We're so much more than these wretched vessels that we sprint or swagger or lurch or limp around in. . . .

Judging from the 175 readers' responses to this article, agreement with these opinions is overwhelming. The columnist has expressed a basic attitude that pervades our culture.

Of course we can transcend our bodies and we can indeed see far beyond the flesh of our bodies. In this chapter we will see, however, that it is our bodies themselves that do this transcending and visioning, through the thoroughly biological organ that is our brain, and not some out-of-body mentality or spirit that hovers above and away from our fleshly selves. In saying this, we are availing ourselves of scientific knowledge. As we shall see, this knowledge does not debase our mind and spirit, but rather increases our amazement and appreciation of our bodyselves.

---

1. Bruni, "These Wretched Vessels," 2012.

EARTHY BODIES ... EVOLUTION WITHIN US

Hebrew Scriptures depict humans as creatures of the earth—when God breathed on earth, the first man was formed, and the very name of that man, "Adam," means "earth." Others say that we are "stardust"—formed from matter that originated in the cosmic Big Bang billions of years ago. In broad strokes, these images convey the same basic picture that has become a main feature of our worldview today. Science reinforces this theme in *fortissimo*; it is in fact the single most forceful message that science delivers to us about what it means to be human. This is the scientific "take" on who we are.

Science brings home to us in unambiguous terms the fact that our selves are *bodyselves*. I may believe, for good reasons, that I am more than science can tell. I will insist, as surely everyone does, that some of the most important and treasured dimensions of my most intimate self are beyond scientific description. But I cannot ignore the fact that what science reveals to us is basic to my selfhood, and if I seek wholeness, science must be integrated with all the rest of what I know and feel about myself.

If we are to know our bodies, we have to understand this scientific message and let it sink deeply into our awareness. Science tells a story that is earthy to the core. Thanks to the scientific accounts we have more knowledge of ourselves today than at any time in human history—and it is body-knowledge, because that is the focus of science. The scientific picture provides enormous and meticulous detail, filled in by the results of innumerable specific studies. You might say that modern science throws light on who we are by showing us what that original stardust, our earthiness, really is—how inexhaustibly many-splendored and complex it is. In many instances, this detailed knowledge can be put to uses—in medicine, for example. The awesomeness of the sciences of the body is something to appreciate and reflect on. The usefulness of that science reminds us that it truly does make a difference. Our religious traditions tell us that in all their richness the dust and stardust are first of all God's dust. But that part of the story is reserved for a later chapter.

"CHRISTIANITY MOST MATERIAL"

William Temple, Archbishop of Canterbury (1942–4), wrote in his Gifford Lectures, *Nature, Man and God* (1934), that "Christianity is the most avowedly materialistic of all the great religions."[2] He understood, as D. R. G. Owen has observed, that

> Christianity teaches that the whole natural, physical order is God's creation and, as such, is both real and good. It is not something from which man is destined one day to escape. And it is not only the Christian doctrine of creation but also the Christian doctrines of the incarnation, the resurrection of the body, and Christ's return to the earth at the end, that make us take the physical order seriously, recognizing that it has an eternal place in God's purposes.[3]

Temple emphasized the significance of the earthy, material order for Christian faith—particularly in the face of versions of the faith that were world-escaping; he was attacking with full force the dualisms between spirit and matter, spirit and nature, humans and nature. Temple's contemporary, the great twentieth-century-priest-scientist Teilhard de Chardin, carried the point still further in his view of the intimate interaction between humans and evolution. He said that we are "evolution become aware of itself," he underscored that we are embodied, not only in the material of earth, but also in its processes of unfolding—its evolution.[4] Nature shapes us and makes us who we are. Teilhard is speaking of the fullness of nature, from the elementary particles, atoms, and molecules of its physical constituents onwards through biological and cultural processes, including what we call mind, spirit, and soul. Embodied in the chemical combinations that became life (single-celled at first, then ever more complex), making its passage in the bosom of earth through processes that produce the biological stuff and winnow it in give-and-take with the surrounding ambience, some genetic variants surviving in the competition for resources, avoiding illness and accident, while others are eliminated. Very infrequently, mutations facilitate a lucky breakthrough here and there that enables a useful novel form to emerge, while unforeseen events wipe out whole communities or facilitate the success of others. Earth is inside our bodies and outside, shaping us in both ways. A few vivid details from the sciences describe our earthy locatedness. These vignettes do not give us a comprehensive understanding of science, but they do give us the scientific take on our bodies and ourselves.

---

2. Temple, *Nature, Man and God*, § 7.
3. Owen, *Body and Soul*, 22.
4. Teilhard de Chardin, *The Phenomenon of Man*, 220.

Our Bodies Are Selves

EARTHY NATURE INSIDE US

We learn from genetics that earthy nature is inside us. Each of us carries 3 billion nucleotides within our bodies—molecules that structure our DNA and our RNA. They form the nucleic acids that are commonly referred to as A, C, G, and T/U—adenine, cytosine, guanine, and thymine (uracil in RNA). These have been likened to letters, which pair with others to "spell out" our development through the formation of the proteins that constitute our bodies. The nucleotides we have inherited—some from our mother, some from our father—bond with each other to develop our traits and in some cases to bond in faulty ways that cause disease and distortion. My own spina bifida is a direct result of how my ACGT's bonded. This is one fundamental expression of the fact that we are our body chemistry—an ironic twist on the bygone Du Pont slogan: "Better Living through Chemistry." We live by our internal chemistry, which follows its own patterns of evolution. Darwinian processes of evolution are taking place within our very own bodies, from the moment of conception onwards. These processes condition who we are and who we are becoming—in fundamental ways.

The range of scientific approaches to the earthy nature within us is staggering, and it is continually expanding. Nanomedicine, sometimes in concert with bioengineering, is one such approach that is rapidly expanding. The emerging field of synthetic biology belongs in this array of research endeavors; it aims at the design and construction of new biological functions and systems not found in nature. Genetics works at the level of the gene and its constituents, which is very small, smaller than our common sense can even imagine. Nanotechnology and synthetic biology work at that same level. A nanometer is one billionth of a meter; a meter is about 39 inches long. When we speak of nucleotides, as I did earlier, we are in the world 0.3 nanometers. In size, a nanometer compares to a yardstick as a marble compares to planet earth. 25,000 nanometers equal the thickness of a human hair. Genetic engineering manipulates our genes; Nanotechnology works with atoms and molecules, manipulating them to form machines—sometimes called nanorobots or nanobots—that can do important work inside our bodies. Such machines can image the behavior of cells or deliver medication to targeted cells.

The scale of these efforts is so small, but it makes enormous impacts on us by rearranging the building blocks of our bodies—our earthiness—in ways that can cure disease and enhance our lives. The nanosciences and technologies remind us that atoms and molecules, too, are building blocks of our bodily selves. And those building blocks do make a difference—so great a difference, that nanoparticles are widely used to treat cancer every day. When some hospitals advertise that they treat cancer at the "molecular level," it is a sign that they are using nanotechnologies.

A third scientific perspective on our earthy nature is neuroscience, which studies our central nervous system, whose center is our brain. Keep in mind that our brain *is* body—it is a biological organ, just like our other organs. You can hold it in your hand—a quivering mass replete with folds and grooves. But what an extraordinary organ it is! Neuroscience tells us about how our brain is put together (its structure), how it works (its functions), and the difference it makes to how we live our lives. While genetics and bioengineering open up the mind-bending complexity of our bodies, the neurosciences unveil even more. The gray jelly-like mass that fills our skulls has about the same volume as a grapefruit. This "grapefruit" has on the average about 30 billion nerve cells, known as neurons. Neurons communicate with each other through synapses—and each of those neurons may have 10,000 synaptic connections. There are billions of billions of these synapses in our brains—an unimaginable number that may also be used to describe the number of stars in a galaxy. The activities of these billions of nerve cells are now being researched in order to relate them to the activities and traits of our ordinary lives—our ability to move our limbs or use language, for example. Our personality characteristics are also in this mix of brain activity. We'll elaborate more on this later, but such things as our moods, feelings that we "belong" or that we are lonely, for example, are correlated to activities of our brains; they are the subject of the cognitive sciences.

The significance of these scientific research areas becomes clear when we ask what difference they can make for our lives. The diagnostic success of procedures that have been developed in tandem with genetics, nanomedicine, and neuroscience, for example, may lead to prescribing drugs that enable a person immobilized by depression to become an alert, active person who can participate in a community and make a contribution to it—recall the example with which we opened this chapter. On the basis of knowledge about an individual's body, drugs may be tailored specifically for a given person—designer drugs. The diagnostic procedures and the drugs are material interventions derived from knowledge of our thoroughly material bodies—but they make a difference for our personalities, our zest for life, for all the dimensions that we call "personal" and "spiritual."

We need to underscore that the scene of action in these myriad processes within us is *our bodies*. Even when the outcomes involve our minds and spirits, the interface is body. The genetic evolution and manipulation impinges on our bodies, and the same is true of the activities of those 30 billion neurons and the billions of synaptic connections in our brains. Equally, the bioengineering interventions of synthetic biology and nanotechnology are through and through transactions of our bodies, in our bodies. Our bodies, wrapped in their skin, are the theater of this action—we meet the world within our skin on bodily terms.

. . . IN AN EARTHY WORLD—EVOLUTION OUTSIDE US

It is this same body, wrapped in this same skin, which meets the world outside us. We might picture sardines tightly packed together in a can—so bodily engaged are we with earthy nature all around us, as close as the air we breathe and as distant as the formation of the universe. There is no distance whatsoever between us and this nature. Sardines in a can is one way to image this closeness between us and the nature around us; we think also of images of being clothed, of being wrapped in it, or bathed in nature. As I cited him earlier, Teilhard wrote of the material world that "we find ourselves so surrounded and transfixed by it, that there is no room left to fall down" and contemplate it.[5] We are not just inhabitants of this earthy nature that is outside us, nor simply formed from it as depicted in the second chapter of Genesis, when God breathed spirit into the clay. This skin we inhabit is a permeable membrane. We interpenetrate it, and it reciprocates. The air we breathe becomes part of us, and so does the water. The food we consume merges with our cells, nourishing them and also polluting on occasion. We are, literally, what we eat. The world outside transmutes into an inside world, as well. This outside/inside dance with our world takes thousands and thousands of permutations, but an example or two brings it home to us.

Let's begin with the natural world at a distance, the cosmic processes that occurred billions of years before our planet even existed. The evolving of the cosmos for example had to be long enough in time for a planet to appear that possesses atmosphere and other conditions congenial for life to emerge. Those 7 to 8 billions of years that it took for the universe to provide conditions congenial to our planet and its life may seem irrelevant

---

5. Teilhard de Chardin, *The Divine Milieu*, 83.

to our lives, but in fact without their evolution, we would not be here today. Divine creation may be the source of our life on earth, but God took this long evolutionary route to make us. It takes this long to make human bodies. Furthermore, several elements that were formed in the universe before there was a planet earth are essential for human life today—the fluoride for our teeth and iron in our blood are just two examples. The history of the universe does make a difference for us.

We skip ahead several billion years to the Age of the Dinosaurs, 136 million years ago (mya). Robert Bakker provides a stunning insight into an aspect of this dance in his 1995 "dinosaur novel," *Raptor Red*. In one scene, the actors are one "aegi," a tiny shrew-like mammal whose Latin name is *Aegialodon dawsoni*, and an ostrich dinosaur, also known as an ornithomimosaur, who is thought to have resembled ostriches and to be bird-like. This dinosaur weighed as much as a rhino, stood sixteen feet tall, and its arms had a reach of over eight feet. There is a backstory to the scene Bakker describes: when they flourished, the dinosaurs very effectively went after small mammals as tasty prey. Since we humans emerged in the mammal line, it is fair to say that our existence was dependent on one of two occurrences, either the mammals eluded the dinosaurs or the dinos became extinct before they ate all the mammals—or, as seems to have happened, both of these came to pass.

Bakker, who has devoted his life to searching for dinosaur fossils and studying them, provides a priceless fictional scene of how mammals may have eluded their predators.

> The big ostrich dino hen drives all six claws down hard. They come up holding a wriggling piece of prey.
>
> She flips the little body into the air.
>
> Gulp!
>
> "Yeaccch"
>
> It's a frog. There's nothing wrong with frogs for brunch, but she was expecting the taste of furball. Oh, well, one gulp is as good as another.
>
> Still, she pauses a minute thinking, *I grabbed a furball—tossed it—it became a frog. Never saw that happen before.*
>
> If she were interested in metaphysics, she might invent the first dinosaur religion then and there. Instead, she moves on, hunting, digging, and gulping.
>
> *Aegialodon* the scorpion-killer stays absolutely still. He's survived and he'll live to a ripe old age—eleven months. By that time his aegi genes will be in swarms of children and grandchildren.

Our Bodies Are Selves

Over a hundred million years later, the flow of aegi of genes will produce wonderful creations—giraffes, elephants, rhinos, whales, bats, monkeys, chimps, Democratic senators, Republican majority leaders. Charles Darwin himself. All can be traced back to the supreme bug popper, the *Aegialodon*.[6]

This scene is fanciful, of course, but it retrieves in a whimsical manner the material conditions in which the evolutionary process took the twists and turns that may have made our very existence possible. Notice how material and earthy this process is—a very appropriate reminder of how the stuff of the earth makes us who we are.

Under the chapter heading, "Two-Tiered Drama," Bakker gives us the backstory for the episode that he has just recounted:

> At this moment, on that Early Cretaceous day, a double-level drama is being played out. On top of the stage made by the ground surface, raptors and acros play the leading roles of large and super large predators. Below the stage, underground, another storyline is being played out, by a supporting cast of tiny creatures who shun the daylight.
>
> If you are the size of mouse, a frog is a grotesque monster from a fairy tale. The Aegialodon is only a one-ounce insectivorous Cretaceous furball, a twitchy lump of hard muscle, long snout, beady black eyes, exquisitely sensitive whiskers, and spreading five-clawed feet fore and aft. A frog face has appeared in the aegi's burrow. The frog's mouth is almost wide enough to swallow the aegi.
>
> The frog had been crouching near the aegi's burrow, only to be pushed into it by a running dino hen who narrowly missed stepping on the frog.[7]

These are scenes of evolution in action—as such they do not provide a comprehensive understanding, but rather they are representative snapshots. We took one snapshot from the origin of our universe—12 billion years ago—and another along the pathway of life's evolution, from the Age of the Dinosaurs, known in scientific terms as the Cretaceous Period (136 million years ago). These time spans, millions and billions of years, are dizzying when we try to comprehend them. Our third snapshot jumps ahead to our early ancestors, 41,000 years ago. It may help us to understand these time periods to recall that the most famous cave paintings, the Lascaux

---

6. Bakker, *Raptor Red*, 155.
7. Ibid., 137.

paintings, date from about 30,000 years ago and the beginnings of agriculture from 10,000 years ago.

Imagine that the history of the universe is put on a twelve month calendar, with one day equaling 33 million years and 1 hour equaling one and one-third million years. By this reckoning, the dinosaurs appear on the day after Christmas, and our next snapshot, which deals with our early human ancestors, would occur during the last minute before the cosmic clock strikes midnight. This imaginative way of depicting the timeline of our universe's history is important as a reminder of just how late in the game human beings emerged and how much history has prepared the way for our moment. Apparently, God was doing a great deal *before* we were created, and chose a stupendously complex and arduous process to bring us into being. This awareness by itself, is enough to persuade us that in these matters—no matter how much scientific knowledge we have, and no matter how exciting it is—we are dealing with mystery. Our understanding of ourselves and how we came to be what we are, as well God's purposes for doing it this way—all is wrapped in mystery.

Now we view our third snapshot of the evolutionary journey that our bodies have taken. This picture of our journey was not available before March 2010, when a collection of bones was discovered in a cave in the Siberian Altai Mountains. Scientists discovered that the cave had been inhabited by modern humans (sometimes called Cro-Magnon), Neanderthals, and a third group, named Denisovans (after the name of the cave), who up to this time had not been recognized as a distinct species. The bones, dated 41,000 years ago, were subjected to DNA analysis. This analysis revealed an exciting result: the three groups had not only lived in the cave, but they had formed bonds and interbred. Up to 17 percent of the Denisovan DNA is of Neanderthal origin, while up to 6 percent of the modern human DNA originates with the Denisovans, which is about the same as modern humans. Research is moving quickly in this field, and there are suggestions that additional human groups may be involved. One of the most interesting suggestions from this scientific research is that the DNA from Neanderthals and Denisovans may have contributed significantly to modern human immune systems. Since other species had been in Europe for a longer time, they may well have the developed immune strategies that would enable modern humans to flourish even after Neanderthals and Denisovans (and other possible groups) became extinct.

What does this vignette tell us about our bodies? It gives us a deeper and exciting insight into what makes up this "dust of the earth" or stardust, if you will, from which we have been created. It tells us something about the journey—the struggle, even—that our bodies have taken to reach their present destination.

BIG NATURE AND BIG HISTORY

Nowhere is the mandate to adopt an explosively large concept of nature more evident than when we look at ourselves, human beings who have emerged in a natural history that is millions of years long. This idea of "big history" is gaining currency today; it is included in many high school curricula today.

These vignettes from the distant history of our evolution deal with how we got to where we are. The point is that our life is totally dependent on the processes of natural evolution. Whether we believe that God created us or that nature did, this is the way we were fashioned—through the twists and turns, the zigs and zags of evolutionary processes. The fact that we came through the evolutionary process (represented here by the story of the *aegi*) and that we share the genes from previous stages of life—with the Denisovans and the Neanderthals, for example—reminds us that we are kin to all of life on this planet. This genetic heritage has made us what we are, and it lives within us at this very moment.

The consciousness has grown among us that we are dependent on the nature around us—the air, the soil, the waters—in such ecological images as our dwelling in nature, nature as the house in which we live. We must now develop the awareness of kinship, that we not only live in nature, but that nature lives in us and constitutes our very being. Ecological images can depict external relationships—close, necessary, but nevertheless external. Kinship images are images of internality—nature as it has evolved is literally bone of our bone and flesh of our flesh. And this closeness of ecology and kin focuses on our bodies.

Some people believe that this evolutionary picture is too little and that it diminishes God. Others, to the contrary, argue that evolution makes God unnecessary. For my part, I believe that evolution opens a window on God. We need a big picture of both God *and* nature. To understand how life exists at all, let alone creatures like us, we must have an expansive idea of nature. Scientific and naturalistic descriptions are not enough to account for the wonders of evolution—from Big Bang to *Homo sapiens*. To make sense of this mind-boggling happening, we need a vision of God that is big enough to encompass that trajectory, as well as a huge vision of the incredible possibilities of nature. As Joseph Sittler has written, we need to understand God and God's grace in ways that can swing in the vast orbit of what we know about our universe. Biblical scholar J. B. Phillips wrote a book with the title, *Your God Is Too Small!*[8] We need a comparable admonition, *Your Nature Is Too Small!* The world of evolutionary science calls out for a big nature. Evolutionary science cries out as well for the dimension of depth—where both religion and spirituality come into play. Our times call for large concepts of both God and nature.

Science so successfully unfolds the inexhaustible depths of nature—the "dust of the earth"—that we are compelled to conclude that this dynamic dust is sufficient for the fullness of our bodyselves. With the act of breathing into the earthy loam, God in effect said, "There, that's all that is needed." The Creator could take Sabbath, the work was completed. Later on in this chapter, we will reflect on the meaning of these words, "That's enough."

THE ABCs OF EVOLUTIONARY THEORY

Before we go further let's turn to a more matter-of-fact exposition of what we mean by the term "evolutionary science." There is so much talk about evolution—and controversy—that we need to be clear about how we are using the term in this book. You might say that in the next few pages we will turn to the chalk board to chart some *x*'s and *o*'s from evolutionary science's playbook.

Evolution has not only proven to be enormously successful in guiding research, it has also given rise to a large picture of human beings that is fundamental to our thinking today—it is basic to our worldview. It has been called one of the greatest intellectual achievements of all time, regardless of culture; every attempt to understand human life, whether philosophical or religious, must come to terms with evolution. We cannot hope to understand our bodies and our bodyselves apart from the picture evolution it provides. Evolutionary science is a powerful engine driving the quest for a new paradigm of body.

---

8. Phillips, *Your God*.

Evolutionary science portrays human beings as the products of a long process, that continues today. There are several basic elements in this picture of humans, some of which we have already discussed:

The process is very long—as old as planet earth itself, and even as old as the universe, since life on earth is formed by cosmic events that stretch back to the Big Bang, 12–15 billion years ago (bya). It is more convenient to think in terms of the earth and its evolution of 4.5 billion years, remembering that life appeared on earth 2 billion years ago. Cosmic processes are definitely relevant, however. As with all evolutionary processes, our development is governed by natural laws, but also open to chance.

We are fully embedded in the processes of earth itself. We are not creatures "in" or "on" the planet—we are rather a component of the earth's own processes of development. Teilhard de Chardin said it in a few words: "Humans are evolution-become-aware-of-itself."[9] He also said that we are physically and chemically the most active layer of the earth, the leading edge, the "thinking edge" of our planet. This sense of ourselves is not widely understood, and it is part of the paradigm shift in thinking that we call for in this book.

The process is fully material and natural. There is no intervening force required for the events of evolutionary history to unfold. Each stage of evolution is conditioned by what has gone before, even as it exhibits freedom and surprising developments. Both freedom and determinacy are evident as evolution unfolds. As we will discuss more fully, all that makes us who we are—our brains, minds, feelings, and ideas—is rooted in the material of our bodies.

Context-environment. What we become in our development is elicited by our environmental context. We possess a wide range of genetic possibilities, our *genotype*, but many of them are not actualized. Our actual form is our *phenotype*, and it is dependent upon what fits with our environment. For example, on the average, each of us possesses several lethal genes, but they remain unexpressed unless they are matched by our mate or other factors in the context in which we develop. The phenotype is our body, one of the innumerable printouts of our genotype/genome that are possible. Those printouts are possible phenotypes. The term *epigenesis* makes this point in its insistence that an organism

---

9. Teilhard de Chardin, *Phenomenon of Man*, 220.

does not develop simply according to the preformed plan contained in its genes; rather the entire cell and the environment provide inputs that shape development. For example, working out produces more muscle cells because the workout lifestyle influences gene expression.

Selection. The environment poses a challenge that determines survival—offspring must survive into the next generation. The survival test may apply to individual genes, to individual organisms, and to groups and an entire species. This is called selection—"natural selection," because it is the process of nature itself that selects. The traditional designation of this process as "survival of the fittest" can be misleading, because popular imagination tends to think of "fitness" as physical toughness and bellicosity, as in the phrase, "red in tooth and claw."[10] In fact, fitness may refer also to resistance to disease or ability to compensate for scarce food resources or producing many offspring. "Inclusive fitness" refers to success in producing offspring that flourish. Inclusive fitness is the chief evolutionary criterion of survival.[11]

Evolutionary science is based on a paradigm of recent origin that is still in a dynamic state of expansion and elaboration which includes both the theory of evolution and the actual research that the theory guides and interprets. The theory that undergirds evolutionary science is a comprehensive net of explanatory concepts that is generally associated with the work of Charles Darwin, whose *Origin of Species* first appeared in 1859. Darwin's theory remains fundamental to this day, even as it has been expanded and revised.

A most notable expansion, known as the "modern synthesis," or neo-Darwinianism or neo-Darwinian theory, resulted from the integration of genetics, based on the breakthrough work of Gregor Mendel, whose work was contemporary to Darwin's, even though it was unrecognized until the turn of the twentieth century. The synthesis was worked out in the 1930s and 40s by the work of a number of brilliant biologists, including R. A. Fisher, Theodosius Dobzhansky, Ernst Mayr, and George Gaylord Simpson. Their work brought together ideas from several biological fields: genetics, including population genetics, cytology, morphology, paleontology, and others.

In the last half-century, as the biological sciences have burgeoned, so has the work of expanding and reinterpreting Darwin's work, with the

---

10. Alfred Lord Tennyson, "In Memoriam A. H. H.," canto LVI, line 15.
11. Hamilton, "Evolution of Altruistic Behavior," 354–56.

result that the net of evolutionary concepts has grown vastly in breadth and complexity. Many fields of research have been brought to bear and unified, including: molecular biology, evolutionary developmental biology ("evo-devo"), game theory, paleontological ideas of "punctuated equilibrium," microbiology, epigenetic inheritance, and more. This broad net guides research and interprets knowledge of virtually every aspect of our world and of human beings. Evolutionary theory has become the dominant worldview in our time.

THE PRACTICE OF MEDICINE—MANAGING THE EVOLUTION OF OUR BODIES

We can get a vivid picture of how important evolutionary science has become by looking briefly at the practice of medicine, the social sciences, and the sciences of the "inner self." At the same time, this will fill out our understanding of what science tells us about our bodies and our selves.

There is no need to elaborate on the significance of the practice of medicine in our lives today. At 18 percent it constituted nearly one-fifth of United States gross national product for 2012; the facilities and institutes involved in medical sciences, practice, and healthcare delivery are the largest part of many of our finest universities; healthcare policy has been near the top of public discussion and political process in the U. S. in recent years. The theory of evolution and the research that theory undergirds stand at the very center of this massive concentration on medical practice and healthcare delivery.

As the subtitle indicates, the practice of medicine is our attempt, through our learning and the technical means we have developed, to manage our evolved nature—and even to redirect it in important ways. Most of this medical development is aimed at curing disease or rendering it less lethal—to combat and compensate for the life-threatening factors we were born with or that have beset us in the course of our lives.

It has become a commonplace for us to believe that we can reshape our bodies from head to toe, and even reformulate what goes on inside our bodies—our body chemistry, for example. We need not settle for the bodies we were given at birth—so the thinking goes. This belief comes as welcome news for many, since much of our effort in this direction is necessitated by very serious physical issues: reproductive technologies, cancer therapies, repair for lost limbs, casualties of war, and serious birth defects. Some of our efforts are, to be sure, motivated by vanity and social fads. For example, in 2012, Americans spent $10.4 billion on a total of 14.6 million cosmetic surgery procedures.[12] Approximately 1.6 million of these procedures dealt with serious medical issues, while 13 million were of a more trivial, "minimally invasive" nature.

Our practice of medicine makes it clear—more vividly than almost any other area of life—how dependent we are on our bodies and how much we rely on scientific knowledge and expertise to keep our bodies functioning. What we see here is evolutionary knowledge and skill turning back upon themselves to alter the course of evolution within our bodies. Research into the nature of AIDS gives us a clear example of this. In order to develop effective treatments against the disease, it was necessary to study and understand the very complex evolutionary processes by which the virus develops and defends itself against attack. When these processes were understood, it was possible to develop strategies that can go counter to the virus's evolved behavior and penetrate its defenses.

THE SOCIAL SCIENCES: THE EVOLUTIONARY ECOLOGY OF HOW WE BEHAVE

The biologist Edward O. Wilson published his landmark book, *Sociobiology*, in 1975.[13] Almost immediately, it unleashed a storm of protest, because it aimed at delineating the biological bases of all animal behavior, including the behavior of humans. Although sociobiology solidified and extended the work of many scientists, across a number of fields, it elicited a wave of criticism, particularly from the social sciences—psychology, sociology, and anthropology—as a program that would reduce human beings to their biological nature. Wilson was charged with the attempt to "biologicize" the social sciences.[14] He and his cohorts responded that their goal was to uncover the biological dimension of human behavior and integrate it into our understanding of humans.

The intervening years have supported the program of sociobiology. It is now quite in the mainstream to speak of the biological *and* cultural evolution of humans, and thus the term *biocultural* evolution has come into vogue. In nearly every university, the departments of psychology, sociology,

12. American Society of Plastic Surgeons, "2012 Plastic Surgery Statistics Report," 5.
13. Wilson, *Sociobiology*.
14. Wilson, *Naturalist*, 130–54.

or anthropology, include studies of the genetic and evolutionary components that relate to the field. The term *sociobiology* itself has fallen victim to the critical turmoil, however, and we are more likely to encounter the term, "the ecology of human behavior."

In psychology, it is commonplace to take account of the relevant genetic factors of our psychological makeup and behavior, as well as the evolutionary history of the phenomena under study. Some researchers in the field go so far as to ally themselves with the discipline called "evolutionary psychology," while many others simply pursue this research without attaching any label to it. John Cacioppo's work on loneliness and social connection is a prime example. In his book, *Loneliness: Human Nature and the Need for Social Connection* (2008), Cacioppo puts human behavior in a meticulously delineated biological and evolutionary context.[15] He also employs the work of cognitive neuroscience. Much of psychiatry has also adopted this approach, using psychotropic drugs to manipulate the processes that are thought to be at the root of mental illness.

Research in anthropology, in a widespread fashion, includes the perspective of "biocultural anthropology," which is still distinguished in some circles from "cultural anthropology." William Irons has been a proponent of the biocultural approach for many years—as exemplified by his studies of the evolution of morality and religion.[16] Primate studies have been a rich field for relating our evolutionary history to current human behavior, particularly in the work of Richard Wrangham[17] and Frans de Waal.[18]

The contributions of sociobiology to sociology have been mixed, but many sociologists agree with the research of Francois Nielsen and Gerhard Lenski that provides essential knowledge into sex and gender roles, the theory of collective action, and the elaboration of a richer and more complex model of human nature. Biologist Richard Alexander's work, *The Biology of Moral Systems,* is such a contribution, showing how an evolutionary perspective illuminates the emergence of morality as a social behavior and the various social purposes it has served.[19]

---

15. Cacioppo and Patrick, *Loneliness*.

16. Irons, "How Did Morality Evolve?" 49–89.

17. Wrangham, "The Evolution of Social Structure," 282–96; and Wrangham and Peterson, *Demonic Males*.

18. Frans de Waal, *Good Natured*; and Frans de Waal, ed., *Tree of Origin*.

19. Alexander, *The Biology of Moral Systems*.

MAKING SENSE OF THE SCIENCE

What does all this amount to? We can state it briefly: our humanness is thoroughly and completely embodied, both in its external relationships, in the worlds in which we have emerged and now live our lives, and in the most interior recesses of our personalities. The evolutionary sciences have crossed the frontier into our inner life. The neurosciences, which focus on the brain, working within the evolutionary paradigm, play into the understanding of the psychology and the wider evolutionary history that makes us who we are. How we imagine ourselves, how we relate to other people, even our most intimate inner thoughts and feelings—all of this is illuminated by understanding the evolutionary past in which we have emerged and the ways that past shapes our present moments.

Some may say that this reduces us and our lives to natural processes, that it makes our humanity a lesser thing, and that it quenches our human spirit. Such a response misses the point. We are not "reduced" at all—rather, our nature and the nature that has allowed us to emerge become much more wonderful, profound, and even more of a mystery. The sciences, as we have surveyed them in a few illustrative vignettes, underscore and throw light on what it means to be embodied—to be bodyselves. When we speak of our human spirit, our creativity, imagination, our care and love for others; when we speak of ourselves as God's created persons, living in the wider creation that God has brought forth—all of this is testimony to what nature, and our embodiment in nature, can become and are destined to become under the creative caring of God.

8

The Human Journey

Philip Hefner

CLEARLY, WHEN WE SPEAK of bodies, we are speaking of ourselves, and furthermore our bodies as they are embedded in technology. Rather than thinking of ourselves as abstractions, our selves are a rich mix of dimensions that defy separation—they exist together in ways that our words and concept struggle to understand. The central issue is human identity. It's about the struggle to arrive at the meaning of being human today, or theological anthropology. The struggle to arrive at human meaning is the grappling with our own human creativity, particularly in its technological expression. This struggle is at the heart of our being today; it grows out of our very nature as we try to discern the future of our culture.

This chapter presents another "take" on our bodyselves—a natural outreach for our thinking, even as it extends far beyond the scope of this book.

A note about terminology is in order. We commonly talk about "human being," but this can be confusing. The word "being" is both a noun and a verb form. It can refer to us as creatures, members of the species *Homo sapiens*. So, we can say, "She is a human being." It also refers to the activity of *being* human. So, we can say, "Human *being* is a challenge to us," which means the same as "*Being* human is a challenge to us."

Both "being human" and the "human being"—are a process, a *becoming*. Human beings could just as well be referred to as "human becomings." We are "becomings." We are caught up in the process of human becoming, and we are struggling to understand what it means to become human.

WE ARE WRITING A PERSONAL NARRATIVE, A MEMOIR

What kind of venture is this, which describes its theme as "becoming human?" We can grasp its meaning in terms of "memoir." We are all writing our own memoir.

What is memoir? Vivian Gornick offers an explanation.[1] Memoir is not fiction, neither poetry nor novel nor a piece for the theater. It must be creative, to be sure, but it is not fiction. Memoir is not journalism or science. It does not presume to be so detached in its objectivity that it simply reports some truth "out there," with no personal involvement for the writer. Memoir is not just the facts. Nor is memoir autobiography, in which it is perfectly acceptable, as Gornick says, to fall "into the pit of confessionalism or therapy on the page or naked self-absorption."

In contrast, the memoir describes a situation—my situation, our situation—and tells a story that makes sense of the situation. One facet of our situation is our genes and culture. Humans as creators and technological crisis are coordinates that map our situation. Journalism and science can place the situation at center stage and put the sense of meaning of that situation aside. Fiction, on the other hand, can take liberties—poetic license we call it—in describing both situation and its possible meaning. Autobiography, for instance, can focus entirely on what happened to me and how I reacted to it.

Memoir must take a different tack. What makes a compelling memoir is a credible description of its author's situation, as well as a clear sense of the self who struggles in that situation. Further, it is the forging of an interpretation that can respond to the "So What?" question of the self in the situation—an interpretation that grapples with the meaning of the self's entanglement in its situation. When we speak of memoir, we are dealing with what Gornick also calls *personal narrative*.

What do religion and science have to do with memoir and personal narrative? They have everything to do with it, because science is a fundamental element of our situation today, and religion is challenged to tell a

---

1. Gornick, *The Situation and the Story*.

story that will make sense of that situation. There is more to our situation than science, but there is very little in our situation today that does not have a thread of connection to science and its consequences. Each one of us is challenged to tell the story that offers the sense of our situation. Not all of us will bring religion into this story, but many of us will. In this respect the religious effort is part of the larger human effort to discern meaning. Whether religious or not, we are comrades, brothers and sisters together writing our personal narrative in the attempt to make sense of our situation.

Memoir reminds us that the sense we are looking for is not abstract, far removed or "other" from us; it is the meaning of ourselves that we are after. Each of us and all of us together are engaged in this personal narrative. When we struggle for our own meaning, it is then that a new awareness of our situation dawns on us. This new awareness becomes our principal statement about our situation. We are discovering—it is being revealed to us—that our experience in the world is moving us toward new understandings and interpretations of who we are. We are in the process of discovering that we are indeed caught up in a process of becoming that requires fresh ideas, fresh images of ourselves. The images of us as creators and as created co-creators are emerging in this process of self-discovery.

BOTH CREATED AND CREATOR?

A sense is emerging that we are creators, by our very nature and experience. However, we are as much creat*ed* as creator. The scientific story tells us that the processes of nature have created us, by means of evolution. We did not give ourselves our physical-chemical-biological composition, nor did we give ourselves brains and the culture that they make possible and necessary. When we turn to our religious traditions, we will see that they speak of our being created by God. These natural processes that have engendered us are declared to be the instrumentality of the divine Creator.

Since we are created as we are, the conclusion to be drawn is that we are *created* creators. There is linkage, however, between the source of our being created and our own creativity. I try to capture the fullness of this linkage by using the term, "created co-creator." To the degree that evolving nature has created us, our own creating is taken up into that nature, so that we are nature's own creators, co-creators with the evolutionary process that has engendered us. If we view ourselves as created by God, as the religious traditions tell us, we are God's co-creators.

We find ourselves in a strange situation. We are aggressive, forward looking, intent on making plans and carrying them out. But we are finding that in our aggressiveness, we are on the receiving end of a process that we did not plan or even foresee. We sense that we are undergoing transformations that do not fit with our accepted self-images, our received interpretations of what it means to be human. This is truly our situation—in which we are becoming human in ways that we cannot ourselves easily comprehend or take the measure of. And once this awareness dawns on us, we recognize that this process of becoming did not begin just yesterday—it has been years, decades, even millennia in the works. We did not know it, because we had to discover it. Once we begin to discover it, we have to forge the ideas that can interpret it for us and tell what its meaning is. We are attempting to tell a story that makes sense of our situation and journey. This is the stuff of memoir.

WHO IS THE MEMOIRIST?

The author of this narrative is you, me, all of us. What is being said, what is being narrated, is the journey of awareness that we are becoming different beings, new beings who cannot be contained by older ideas of who we are. We require new images and ideas that are up to the task of telling us who we are becoming.

A memoir requires a clear sense of the self, of the "we" whose voice inhabits the personal narrative. We who are caught up in this journey of becoming are not abstract ciphers; we are not faceless members of some massive horde. What must we say about ourselves, we who are memoirists of human becoming? Here I lay down a few basic points.

We first of all recognize that we are somewhat off-balance and unsure. We are ourselves undergoing transformations whose end we cannot see: we are caught up in a process of discovery. Our journey of becoming is not a trip to the grocery store with a prearranged list of items to guide us from one aisle to the next, nor it is like a business meeting that we chart ahead of time with an agenda in one hand and Robert's Rules of Order in the other. A better image is that of a driver in a car racing along the interstate highway at seventy miles an hour with a map in one hand, to find the destination, and a service manual in the other, to diagnose and repair defects in the car at the same time. This is our vulnerability, and it is intrinsic to our nature as co-creators.

VULNERABILITY AND AMBIVALENCE

We write our narrative out of our vulnerability in this situation—little wonder that we are also anxious writers. We are ambivalent. On the one hand, we are eager to reach our destination, but, on the other, we are not happy at the prospect of our own ignorance as to where that destination lies and what the conditions of the highway are. It is not always pleasurable for us to undergo transformations that we cannot control or even predict. Our own personal ambivalence is reflected in the larger community and society, because we do not all respond in the same way to the prospect of transformation.

For some of us, the scientific accounts have rendered the religious views unbelievable; scientific understanding has displaced the religious—at least on the surface. Others, contrariwise, are so uncomfortable with the naturalistic accounts of science that they opt for religious interpretations at the expense of science—also at least on the surface. This ambivalence, in my view, is on both sides. The secularists hold on to high valuation of human being that has its roots in our religious traditions, while those who oppose evolutionary interpretations of human being continue to go for medical treatment whose cornerstone is evolutionary biology.

We are also ambivalent about the idea of "human becoming," because we often prefer stable, unchanging states. We often would like to think of human nature as something fixed and reliable. Some believers in the Bible would rather read Genesis 1 as if the theory of evolution had never been formulated. At the same time, a secular thinker like Francis Fukuyama, in his thoughtful book *Our Posthuman Future*, argues that biotechnology is dangerous because it threatens to alter human nature. This is illustrative of our vulnerability in that we are undergoing transformations whose end we cannot see and are often caught up in the process of discovery.

For instance, many people would rather not struggle with new values of life that are engendered by current options in reproductive technology, because they prefer to think of sexuality and procreation as if those technologies had never emerged.

We should not try to hide from ourselves or from the outside world that we the memoirists are off balance, ambivalent, vulnerable, anxious, and caught in the crossfire of differing opinions and values within ourselves. Recognizing this about ourselves is essential for the substance of our personal narrative and for its credibility. In fact, this is what our memoir is about—how we respond to our situation of vulnerability and ambivalence *as well as* how we interpret its meaning.

THE FRAGMENTS

Finally, we recognize that even though we seek the largest meaning possible for our personal narrative, we access that larger meaning through fragments. Saint Paul recognized this when he said that we see through a glass darkly (1 Cor 13:12, KJV). God as the voice out of the whirlwind told Job very clearly that his understanding was fragmentary (Job 38:1—40:2 and 40:6—41:14).

Jews, Christians, and Muslims among us will want to bring God into the memoir. These three religions find their common point of contact in Abraham, whose place as a father of faith is grounded in his willingness to devote his life to a journey whose outcome he could not know. He knew God as the one who called him to travel. In Christian traditions, Martin Luther and the Eastern theologians stand out as theologians of fragments. Luther understood that all talk about God was through a glass darkly. He spoke of the hidden God whose nature is known only through the fragment of Jesus Christ and his cross. The Eastern theologians, epitomized in Dionysius the Areopagite, recognized that finally it is not possible to speak about God—this is known as *apophatic* theology. When we do speak about God it is against a background of unspeakableness. Even theologians in the tradition who seemed to speak a great deal about God, such as Augustine, Anselm, and Thomas Aquinas, went to great lengths to remind us that our talk about God is not straightforward and direct, but rather analogical. How could it be otherwise, since God is infinite and our minds are finite?

Science gives us helpful images for this point. Think of our knowledge of the universe and its evolution. We are infinitesimally small creatures on a small planet revolving around one of a billion billion stars. The universe is now so vast that it is not possible to communicate its breadth. We came on the scene at least 12 billion years after the universe got its start, and by most estimates the universe is not even half way through its evolution. Yet we seek the knowledge of this universe, both its present state and its origins and its ending. The image comes to mind of a corpuscle in my bloodstream, or a cell in my body, seeking to understand me, from my conception to my death and everything in between.

We have only fragments for the basis of our knowledge, but the fragments are real. The writer of the memoir knows that the fragment we have is our own life, our own situation, our own journey. The memoirist knows that the only chance of real and trustworthy knowledge requires honest attentiveness to the fragment that is us and that our only chance of discovering the truth is by being faithful to the fragment we have been given—our experience of the journey that is becoming human.

Our journey of becoming human lies through this unexhaustiveness of nature. Job called it the whirlwind, Luther spoke of theology of the cross, Kierkegaard insisted that only indirect discourse is appropriate on this journey. Our personal narrative, our memoir, begins with recognizing that our situation is a fragment, convinced that attention to that fragment and the search for its meaning is not only our best hope, it is the substance of becoming human.

Our memoir must be about the human journey, about the struggle to arrive at the meaning of being human today. It is a journey searching for new symbols by which to interpret an experience that is formative for our times. This journey is also a journey of becoming human. Here we want to examine religion-and-science in this larger context of what it means to become human in our time.

The image of ourselves as creators stands out as a centerpiece of our reflections. There is an emerging image of who we are that is coming from our human experiences, particularly our scientific endeavors and technology. Who we are is not firmly fixed in our minds, is still much debated, and has yet to find a consensus. At the same time, the image is very real. This image is scientific in that it is provoked and undergirded by scientific evolutionary views of human development, but the image is also a matter of common human experience throughout much of the world. However, the scientific understanding and the common experience are brought into the spotlight because of an intense crisis of creativity in which we find ourselves. It often happens this way, that when we are in crisis, in danger of losing what is familiar and valuable to us and also feeling the lure toward unexplored territory, we gain a clarity about ourselves that is lacking in more tranquil times.

Common Experience

Our experience is that we are able to do things that are novel: that we are able to change the world around us and the world within us in ways that seem new. We can test a pregnant woman, determine the condition and genetic development of the life she is carrying within her and contemplate a number of interventions for the sake of mother or unborn child. We can rearrange the molecules of the earth's natural resources to develop new substances, such as nylon, plastics, or synthetic skin and bone. We regularly fabricate life-sustaining environments that enable men and women to travel and work in outer space. We rearrange genetic structures so as to enable goats to give milk that is especially beneficial to humans, or pigs to grow organs that are friendly for transplant to humans. We have created a cyberworld.

Such experiences are not all brand new; some have been available for decades. They point to our experience of imagining and actually creating alternative worlds. We rearrange matter; we can put the pieces of nature's jigsaw puzzle together in unusual ways in order to create new combinations and realities. These experiences reveal our complex and intimate interrelationships with technology—a key part of the story of human becoming we shall explore later. Just as striking as these technological marvels are our imagining and creating of alternative social and political worlds. In my lifetime, for example, I have witnessed the emerging alternative world in which gender roles have been rearranged, as well as the relations between the races. The social world called "family" has undergone transformation, so much so that it is simply no longer possible to impose the older norm of the nuclear family in which a father comes home from work to greet two children who have spent the day under the nurturing care of a stay-at-home mother—that is now one form of family, not the norm. And, of course, I have lived through the era when the socialist and communist movements attempted to reshape entire societies in dramatic ways—and, as in the case of China, have not failed.

At the core of these examples is the experience of ourselves as "creators." These examples flesh out the conviction with which I began telling the human story. Everything I cover here is intended to clarify and interpret this experience. This experience is not tangential to our lives today, not a secondary element, but rather it is central. I believe it is an essential component of becoming human in our present times.

Scientific Perspectives

Scientific understandings throw light on this experience of ourselves as creators; they underscore its essential character. We have evolved as creatures of genes and cultures. I am not suggesting a dualism, as if one could draw a line down our middle and say to one side we are genes, to the other, culture. Furthermore, adaptation to the physical and social environment is a third member of any equation that includes genes and cultures. These are only categories of analysis; in actuality, they are so integral to one another that it is a serious error to think of them in terms of dualism.

To say that we are genes is to acknowledge our physical-chemical-biological constitution as one pathway by which we become human. Physically and chemically, we reveal our ancestry in the galaxies and stars in which the elements of our planet and our bodies originated. We are creatures of stardust, some like to say. Biologically, we declare our kinship with all life forms that emerge in the primal soup, or the primal steam vents, or whatever original conditions are denoted by the various theories of life's origins. In recent years, we have been reminded how much of our DNA we share with chimpanzees, or even with earthworms. Genes speak not only of our constitution and our journey to the position of *Homo sapiens*, they also speak of the present programs that govern so much of our development. In my childhood, I learned that genes programmed eye color; now we know that predisposition to certain illnesses and defects, even moods and personality, have an element of genetic programming. Even our mortality, our growing old and dying, is written into our genetic composition.

Genes are essential, but genes alone do not a human being make. Our evolution has given rise also to a fully biological organ called the brain or central nervous system. The brain is the seat of learned and taught behaviors and the symbols by which we interpret our learning and teaching—that is what we mean here by the term culture. Culture is as essential to us as genes are. If you have watched a calf being born in the barnyard, you may be impressed, as I am, at how quickly, in a matter of minutes and hours, the calf gets to its feet, walks, finds its mother's milk, and gets a start in life. In our contemporary agricultural system, there is, to be sure, some cultural involvement in that calf's birth—the learning and teaching involved in artificial insemination, enhanced feeding, and the like. How different, however, from the birth of my granddaughter a number of years ago. Not only was prenatal medical care necessary for the mother, but father and mother together also took classes in birthing and caring for infants. At each well-baby visit, the doctor not only gives a verdict of "fine" or "needs some special attention," but also a report on the percentile of height and weight into which the baby fits for her age group. A modicum of child development theory is conveyed, so that baby Rory received the optimum stimulation for her developing brain and psyche. If human babies received no more cultural attention than the calf, they would die at an early age. Many babies today are sick and dying because they do receive so little cultural attention. Without the culture, their genes would give out.

Medical centers are a symbol of the intense cultural intervention we exercise through our practice of medicine, aimed at keeping our biology functioning, so that our culture can maintain its quality. What goes on at our hospitals is culture intervening in our biology. And since culture has emerged from biology, the practice of medicine is actually a stage of biology intervening in itself. The calf is a mature adult in little more than a year, whereas human development specialists would say that it takes nearly thirty years today to produce a well-functioning adult human being. It does not take our biology thirty years to grow up; our culture requires the three decades in order to acculturate the person for competent, mature living, which accounts for the importance of universities.

Think back to the experience of ourselves as creators. The popular scientific sketch I have just drawn adds to our experience, in that it clarifies that the component of creativity, of being creators, is written in our biology. Our genes, to be sure, exhibit flexibility and unpredictability, but it is our brains and the development of our culture that is shaped by creativity just as surely as our biology is shaped by prior programming and environment. Our culture—learning and teaching—is as fundamental to us as our genes, but with a far smaller element of prior programming. For instance, I marvel when I read about prehistoric humans. How did they learn which plants and animals were suitable for eating? How did the Maya, for example, come to know that corn is an imperfect food unless it is prepared with the introduction of lime, whereupon it becomes fully nutritional?

Culture evolves, of course, just as biology does, although according to different, non-Darwinian laws. Some years ago, I visited the magnificent Museum of Mining at Bochum in the Ruhr region of Germany. Half of this museum is devoted to the history of mining and the other half to the technology of mining. In the historical exhibits, the cultural evolution is set forth vividly from the prehistoric scraping of the earth to the digging of shafts in the earth to the industrialized mining procedures of the last two to three centuries. The climax comes in the depiction of entire villages being relocated so that the ground beneath them can be mined, only to be replaced when the extraction is completed. The huge machines for these operations not only extract the ore, but also carry out several steps of processing before the ore is loaded on trains for the final manufacture. Our experiences of being creators today may be enabled by our primordial genetic-cultural constitution, but it takes the form that we know today because we stand where we do in the evolutionary development of our cultural capabilities. The exhibits of this museum set forth in striking panorama—from prehistoric scraping to contemporary village-replacement—the capability of our brains to imagine the alternative worlds that we then create by means of our cultures.

THE CRISIS OF TECHNOLOGICAL CIVILIZATION

This leads us directly to the element of crisis, which is the third strand that contributes to the awareness of ourselves as creators. I use the term, crisis of technological civilization. In our contemporary experience, technology is central to what I have referred to as culture. Learned and taught patterns of behavior and the symbols that interpret them are nowhere more prominent and powerful than in our technology. Technology has always been with us, from the times of crude stone tools, to the present. But today we live in a new technological situation that can be described this way: through technology we have superimposed our culture over nearly all the natural systems of our planet. Theologian H. Richard Niebuhr, following Bronislaw Malinowski, spoke of culture as an "artificial, secondary environment, which we superimpose on the natural."[2]

It comprises language, habits, ideas, beliefs, customs, social organization, inherited artifacts, technical processes, and values. The word "artificial" is misleading, but Niebuhr's idea is to the point.

The image that comes to mind is that of the clear plastic overlays that we frequently use. We may place a map upon a table and lay upon that map a clear sheet that depicts the river system of the area, over that a sheet that depicts the hills and mountains, and over that one that depicts the population density or the pockets of air pollution, or the like. The original map is there, underneath it all, but we access the map through the overlays. In some such manner, I see our technology in relation to the natural world. The

2. Niebuhr, *Christ and Culture*, 32.

difference is that we cannot easily remove our technological overlays and return to the original map. Domesticated livestock animals, for example, cannot be instantly return to their pre-human state. The Colorado and Rio Grande Rivers cannot be restored to their prehistoric flows. In nearly every area of the world, it would be impossible for human beings who inhabit our planet to live once again, or be once again, as they were in the 1800s. We speak of globalization, and we must acknowledge that it is unlikely that we could turn back into a preglobalized condition, in which the races and nations would live in isolation from one another. It is unlikely that we could ever resuscitate the identical gender roles that marked the interactions of men and women in the era in which I was growing up.

The examples I cite have become hot issues for debate. They are elements of a crisis after all. I intend no value judgments at the moment, however, just description. The critical point to be made is that sometime within the last fifty years or so we reached the point where the domination of natural systems by human cultural systems became a necessity for human survival. For decades, our technological overlays enabled a decline in the mortality rate and the lengthening of human life—an increase in the population. Now, however, the technological overlay not only *enables* the human population, it is a necessity for the *survival* of that population If we forcibly removed our technological interaction with the rest of nature, millions, even billions, of people around the world would perish.

This describes what I mean by the term technological civilization. What is the crisis? How is it to be defined? We must pause for a moment to consider how our techno-culture works. Technology requires continuous conscious awareness, knowledge, planning, competent operation, monitoring, and evaluation—in short, as philosopher Hans Jonas has put it, it requires constant accountability. Technology does not just happen and go its way on its own, as the calf emerges from the cow's belly and steps out into the barnyard. Every time we flip an electrical switch or turn on our faucets, we should remember how fully dependent the flow of light and water is upon massive amounts of human engineering and operational competence—we often call it infrastructure.

Furthermore our technology must not only work on its own, it must interface with millions of other systems in the natural world. Synchronizing with the environment is an inescapable requirement. The crisis of technological civilization resides in the fact that for all of our knowledge and expertise, we are not fully competent to maintain our secondary environment, nor are we able to interface adequately with the other systems of nature. An example: because of our lack of understanding and foresight, our technological capability to enhance the growth of beef cattle with the use of antibiotics fosters resistance in bacteria that threatens human beings. Here we see the intertwining of lack of competence and the failure of our cultural systems to interface properly with other systems in nature. The bacteria are simply doing what they do very well—evolving, adapting, coping with their environment. We knew this all along, but we did not take it into account. This reminds us that other systems of nature are dynamic, constantly evolving—a characteristic that is difficult for us to engineer continuously into our cultural systems.

Technology is rooted in the intrinsic nature of *Homo sapiens,* it is the work of our culture, the product of our brains, as they go about doing what comes naturally to them, imagining alternative worlds and acting on that imagination. Technology is an overlay upon the other systems of nature and comes as naturally to humans as anything else. It is as natural to us as making honey is natural to bees. Technology is natural in this respect. It is not "artificial," as Niebuhr said. Furthermore, it is a natural expression of our nature as creators. If we are not fundamentally creators, this crisis would not exist. This is truly a civilizational crisis, because if we look carefully, we see that nearly every trouble that we experience today has its origins in our culture and our difficulty in conducting our culture adequately.

The crisis of technological civilization is thus quintessentially a crisis of culture and therefore ultimately a human crisis, the crisis of human creators. The crisis has its origins in that which is our distinctive gift, our highly developed brains and their culture. To say that we are incompetent in the exercise of our culture and inadequately synchronized with the rest of nature is to say that in a significant way we are incompetent to be human, incompetent to exercise our gifts, and that we are indeed out of sync with other systems of nature. The crisis therefore challenges us to understand who we are in the scheme of things, specifically, in the natural world. What is the purpose of culture? How are we to conduct it in accord with its purpose? The crisis presses us to gain a sense of our own identity so that we are enabled to respond to these questions.

As I suggested earlier, crisis is revelatory. When we are in danger, when we are threatened with loss, a shaft of light is thrown on what is essential to us, on what matters most to us. In this shaft of light, we encounter the ambiguity of our own human becoming. We hope as well that this light will point us toward adequate responses to that ambiguity.

9

Nature, Mystery, and God

Philip Hefner

PROPOSING AN IDEA OF NATURE

NATURE IS AN EPIC historical narrative—from cosmic beginnings 13 billion years ago in the Big Bang to the emergence of planet earth, its life forms, and the emergence of humans and our culture. A focus on specific segments of the epic may lose sight of the grand epic narrative, which presents us with unimaginable diversity, from cosmic origins to the molecular structure of life, the amazing gamut of living creatures, primates, and human culture. Our basic assumption is that this is one process, one natural hiMstory—nature's epic. We can speak of it as a drama in several acts—cosmos, biology, ontogeny, culture, and the future of the universe. The Christian theological perspective views all of this as God's epic, as well. Nature's epic is one that God has fashioned and that becomes at the same time God's story—it may be but a portion of God's story, but it is the only story we know. We know of no other work of God that matches God's work of nature. A colossal work it is—13 billion years in time, unimaginably vast ranges of space, unbelievably intricate detail at the micro and nano levels.

What concept of nature could possibly sustain this amazing epic, in both its scientific and its theological breadth? This question looms as a fundamental building block in our efforts to construct meaning.

Before we go further, I offer some of my presuppositions.

1. Our chief concern is our bodies and our bodyselves. Bodies are instances/things of nature; nature is the stage on which bodies have emerged and taken their shape. Mapping this stage will deepen our understanding of our bodies.

2. Our idea of nature will be an opening to our idea of God—if we cannot relate nature to God, we cannot integrate our bodies into our faith.

3. Our knowledge of precisely how God is related to nature is very speculative, due to the inherent limitations of our minds and our experience. The relation of God to the world is one of the most difficult of philosophical problems. It involves relating two things, one of which (the world) we can hardly comprehend because it is so vast and so meticulously put together, the other of which (God) so exceeds our mental capacities and experience that we can only speculate. Classically, theology has recognized this difficulty by reminding us that we can only know God as relating to us, which we view through the lens of the revelation of Jesus Christ. We have no knowledge of God's inner nature and intention. The Cappadocian Fathers of the fourth century said God does not exist in the same sense that everything else exists. This situation is called *apophatic,* i.e., we can speak of God only indirectly, only against the background of what we don't know.

4. The sciences are changing and expanding our view of nature in ways that defy imagination—this is something we often don't give attention to. We cannot go into detail here, but just think how recent our scientific knowledge is; we have increased our knowledge of nature more in the last fifty years than in all of previous human history. Our idea of nature today is not our grandfather's idea of nature! Our view of nature is *expansive* when compared to what people thought before our time. This expansive view makes it possible for us to see ourselves as fully natural. This, in turn, is why humans are a key to interpret the rest of nature. We are what nature can become.

5. The last twenty years have brought a "turn to naturalism." This turn has occurred in the wake of the sciences giving us a picture of nature as incredibly varied and giving birth to the new and unexpected; nature has the capability to be self-creating—more technically called *autopoeisis* or self-generation. Nature defies reductionism. It is boundlessly rich

and constantly producing new things. As a result, today we look first and foremost for natural explanations of everything. Of course, we know that natural explanations cannot account for all that we experience, but we must search for answers within nature before we consider answers outside nature. Naturalistic explanations are the default modes for understanding our world. This may sound reductionist, but I remind you that today we have an expansive view of nature.

6. Nature is so entwined with human activity of molding our world to serve our survival that technology and nature are scarcely distinguishable. Hence the axiom that today nature is technonature.

7. The question of what causes our experience is important. For example, when certain combinations of genes are correlated with such traits as adventuresomeness, others with nurturing and kindness, it is frequently said that genes cause the one or the other behavior. The same kind of search for causes correlates the release of the hormone oxytocin to bonding between persons, sexual activity, trust, generosity, and empathy, leading to the conclusion that oxytocin causes these inclinations; oxytocin has been called the "love hormone." Portions of the brain are associated with specific activities, such as language, or with specific moods, as anxiety or loneliness, with the same conclusions being drawn, that the brain causes the activities or moods.

Such conclusions, sometimes considered to be materialist or naturalist perspectives, are also referred to by the term *nothing-buttery*—love is *nothing but* hormones, anxiety is *nothing but* brain activity. For many of us, however, this *nothing-buttery* is not adequate; we are not persuaded that Shakespeare's plays can be explained by his genome or his brain's activity; brain activity does not explain, for example, Johnny Cash's "Folsom Prison Blues" or Meryl Streep's unforgettable portrayal of Sophie Zawistowski, in the movie, *Sophie's Choice*.[1]

But we are not abandoning the perspective from nature; rather, we present our own take on nature. There is no denying the decisive involvement of genes. Our bodily nature—in this case, our neurobiology or genome—participates fully in our loving and our creating and in everything else that we are and do. My distinctiveness as a person is carried by my equally personal genetic make-up and neurological equipment. But the correlations between the material functioning and structure of body and

---

1. *Sophie's Choice*, directed by Alan Pakula, 1999.

the traits and talents of my personality do not translate into the nothing-buttery of materialist reductionism. *They underscore rather that our body's natural structures and functions are capable, suitable, and fundamental for talking about what we call our "mind" and "spirit."* We might call this an "*ecstatic* naturalism"—that nature has the capacity to step outside itself, to transcend itself, and yet all the while never losing its character as nature. Our bodies, for example, are spiritual and mental and self-transcending at the very same time that they are nothing else but *bodies*. This is not a reductionist perspective, but rather an acknowledgment of the fullness of nature, particularly as its possibilities are progressively unfolded through scientific research. We are adopting a version of philosopher and theologian Nancey Murphy's proposal of "non-reductive physicalism."[2]

This "ecstatic nature" defies final explanation, although we never cease to search for explanations and causes—nor should we. We are compelled to confess and honor the *mystery* of nature—the profound mystery of who we are. For us, this is an opening to talk about God; we believe that an adequate view of nature requires God "in, with, and under" nature, to echo a distinctive Lutheran way of speaking. We contend that such an approach to nature is rooted deeply in the Christian tradition, beginning with the affirmation of the incarnation of God in Jesus and continuing through the centuries in several key teachings and dogmas. Later on, we tie this all together with the idea of a *God-intoxicated* nature.

AN IDEA OF NATURE

Our bodies are occurrences of nature; we *are* nature. How do we begin to think about nature? We deepen our understanding of ourselves by considering nature as the ambience in which our bodies emerge and take shape. R. G. Collingwood, a British philosopher and historian in the first half of the twentieth century, wrote a little book in the early 1940s that has become a classic, *The Idea of Nature*. He emphasized that since nature is so diverse it is impossible to get our minds around it—we crystallize its multiplicity in *ideas of nature*. Nature is a kaleidoscope of shapes, colors, sounds, movements—and creatures. A rushing mountain stream is nature, and so are the water striders that we see walking on the calmer pools nearby and the peaks and forests that surround the scene. And of course, the observer of all this, me for example, is nature, too. It is impossible to grasp the whole

2. Murphy, "From Neurons to Politics—Without a Soul," 357–64.

kaleidoscope in our minds at one time, so we bring it all together in a single idea. The idea is an image that helps us put all the natural forms together. It also forms our understanding and guides our investigations.

According to Collingwood, these ideas do more than focus our understanding of nature; they also determine how we view ourselves and how we relate to everything else. For example, our idea of nature influences whether we consider ourselves to be instances of nature and how we think of our mental and spiritual lives—as well as how we think God relates to nature. As case in point, recall a classic line by Katherine Hepburn in the movie, *The African Queen*.[3] In the movie, Katherine Hepburn plays a missionary in a village in 1914 German East Africa and Humphrey Bogart plays the gin-swilling riverboat captain who delivers supplies to the mission. In one scene, Bogart's character is horrified to discover that Hepburn has tossed all of his bottles of gin into the river. He proceeds to argue with her that it is "only human nature to drink" to which she replies, "Nature, Mr. Allnut, is what we were put in this world to rise above!" In this comment about nature, Hepburn's character reveals how she thought of herself in the world and how she viewed her own body.

Collingwood believed that our ideas of nature have changed over time. The ancient world held to the idea of nature as a living organism, while the Renaissance and Enlightenment viewed nature in analogy to the machine. The twentieth century, under the impact of Darwin's theory of evolution and the quantum revolution in physics, took to the idea of nature as historical process; nature is on a journey, as yet unfinished. In the nearly seventy years since Collingwood wrote, our idea of nature has continued to develop, notably to recognize nature as a realm of emergence. Let us look at this evolving set of ideas in more detail.

All of these ideas—organism, machine, historical process—are linked to experience. (1) *Living intelligent organism*. The ancients experienced nature as permeated by mind; nature is an intelligent living animal and as such it orders itself. The animals inhabiting the earth participate in the world's soul and mind just as they participate in its body. Nature was seen as analogous to the individual human being. (2) *Machine and maker*. Because the Renaissance was preoccupied with new and marvelous machines, think of Leonardo Da Vinci, it is not surprising that they viewed nature through this lens. In contrast with ancient views, they considered nature to be devoid of life and intelligence. Nature's order is imposed by outside forces. The

---

3. *The African Queen*, directed by John Huston.

analogy at work here is a machine and its maker—nature is God's created machine. This view continued to dominate through the eighteenth century. (3) *Historical process.* The sense that reality is historical process or journey is basic to modern experience; it has been said that the nineteenth century invented the worldview or metaphysics of history. Historical studies that placed process, change, and development at the center became the prevailing analogy for an idea of nature. In midcentury, Darwin's evolutionary theories depicted life itself as a developing historical process, and the human species itself had a *natural* history. By the end of the century, scientists were speaking of the physical world in historical terms. Max Planck began by focusing on thermodynamics, and then he and his colleagues spoke of what we now call the "quantum world"—too too small to be seen with the naked eye, in which material things are made up of atoms, which in turn are composed of particles, all of which make their own historical journeys. Philosophers began to speak of reality as *process,* creativity, and the like.

Collingwood's three-stage interpretation of the idea of nature is useful, but we cannot stop where he did, in mid-twentieth century. I suggest three additional elaborations of our idea of nature. (4) *Emergence.* Closely related to the idea of historical process is that of *emergence*—new and unexpected events that seem to come forth from what we see before us without any extraordinary causes that we can detect. They come out of the bottle like the genie, so to speak, and they cannot be put back in as they were before. This experience of the new and unexpected is so basic to our everyday life that we can very well conclude that it is inherent in nature—little wonder that it is also now a significant scientific research item. "Complexity science" is the name that is frequently applied to this research, since novelty seems to emerge in systems composed of interconnected parts that work together in ways that are not predictable if we focus only on the parts individually.[4] The Santa Fe Institute is an example of a scientific effort that devotes itself entirely to complexity/emergence research.[5] The Institute brings together "ideas and principles of many fields—from physics, mathematics, and biology to the social sciences and the humanities—in pursuit of creative insights that improve our world."[6] Their studies include quantum physics, molecular biology, weather, and urban traffic patterns—all of them complex systems in which novelty emerges.

4. Santa Fe Institute, "What Is Complex Systems Research?"
5. http://www.santafe.edu/.
6. Santa Fe Institute, "About."

We still speak of nature as a living organism (think of the Gaia idea) and as a machine (we talk about our heart as a pump and also about our internal "plumbing" or "pipes"), even though these are ideas are really obsolete and misleading. Nature is made up of many organisms; it is not a single super-organism; and there are such things as rocks and volcanoes that are hardly classified as "organic." Viewing our bodies as a machine or an engine may have short-term validity, but we soon discover that our gears and pumps and pipes are living things that do not react like the insides of a watch or an automobile engine. It is still valid to look upon nature as historical process—on a journey, as described by cosmological, biological, and cultural evolution—but the idea of history is not sufficient unless we include that it is a dimension in which surprising new things emerge.

(5) *Mystery.* To these ideas we add yet a fifth that is also deeply rooted in our experience: the idea of mystery. Nature is a realm of knowledge, control, and mystery. (a) Our knowledge about nature, chiefly through our scientific work, is mind-boggling. In the last half-century, we have added millions of pieces of information from dozens of specific sciences to our body of knowledge. Scientific exploration has unfolded a picture of nature—human nature and the larger world—that is mind-bending and inexhaustibly rich. (b) This knowledge has led to our control of nature in ways that we scarcely dreamed of just a century ago. Knowledge has spawned technology that is unimaginably complex and successful in bending nature to our will, from the level of atoms and molecules to that of computers and also earth-moving and space exploration. (c) At the very same time, our knowledge reveals to us how much more there is to know, and our control reveals how successfully nature can defy our attempts to tame it. This is not a question of "gaps" in our knowledge or a breakdown in our control functions. Rather, it is precisely the success of our quest for knowledge and control that makes clear that nature is more than we can comprehend and more than we can ever bring under our control. This awareness brings us to the reality of mystery. Mystery is not a matter of ignorance, not a matter of not knowing enough. Mystery is a matter of richness and texture. One writer speaks of mystery as "the endlessly knowable."[7] Our knowledge about nature continues to grow exponentially, but the more we know about nature, the greater the richness and the deeper the mystery become. This is especially true of our human nature. Theologian Paul Tillich was right when he said that each human being is marked by a mystery, depth, and

---

7. Crowley, "Tomorrow's Theologians," 9.

greatness—and it is enhanced by science. Mystery is a clue to the meaning of our experience of nature.[8]

Consider two examples. For one, the facts of climate change. Our vast knowledge, even in its present imperfect state, enables us to know that climate change is in fact happening and what some of its physical causes are. At the same time, our knowledge tells us that we can understand and control only a small segment of this change—that in large part we must adapt to it where we cannot hope to control it or roll it back. Recall the quite unexpected onslaughts on our East Coast within a six-month period in 2011—record snowfall with 32 inches in Massachusetts alone, a magnitude 5.8 earthquake in Virginia, and Hurricane Irene (the seventh costliest in US history). Attempts to adapt in turn raise questions of human nature and destiny. To what extent can we adapt or not as a human species? How do we make the decisions as to where and for whom adaptive strategies will be made? What are our ethical obligations to those regions and people that will not be able to adapt successfully? What is the human future to be? Is it to be of faith into the unfathomable and unmanageable as we try to make our way?

Or consider the knowledge and control we gain through cognitive neuroscience, through which we trace in detail the brain processes that correlate to such basics as our thinking about specific things (God, for example), our emotions, and our interactions with other people. The detail and complexity of our brain's activity is awesome. This research forms the surface of the even more awesome work of our brains that science does not explain—how these brain processes bring forth a Beethoven symphony or a Bach chorale, a Shakespearean play or a poem by Emily Dickinson, Darwin's theory of evolution or Einstein's theory of relativity, the proposal of Jeffersonian democracy or the Gandhi/King practice of nonviolence. In other words, the amazing scientific charting of our brain's activities exists on the cusp of the richness and mystery of the human spirit. Brain scans do not translate into Beethoven's Ninth Symphony or into a marine's act of heroism in falling on an exploding grenade, thus saving the lives of his comrades, even though the achievements of human spirit are fully embedded in our biology—science intensifies our sense of this embeddedness. The more we know about it, the more we realize that we do not comprehend it—it is mystery. A Benedictine prayer expresses this—"gift us with true humility

---

8. Tillich, "You Are Accepted," 159.

that, in knowing how frail and small we are, we may rejoice even more in the magnitude of your love and the wonders of our own giftedness."[9]

Nature as mystery—we must be clear about how we are using the word. Mystery is not the same as a puzzle. A puzzle can be solved—the more we learn about it and think about it, the closer we come to its solution. Richness and texture characterize mystery. As we dig into it ever more deeply, we come upon ever richer and profounder dimensions of meaning. This endless depth of meaning is not something to be "solved"; it is inexhaustible. So in the example of climate change, we find that over and beyond our increase of knowledge and devising changes in behavior we are engaged with the world of nature in an ongoing quest for understanding our relationship with nature, which in turn brings us face-to-face with questions of human destiny—(1) Just what should we be about in our relations with the natural world? (2) What is the purpose of human behaviors toward nature? (3) What are our obligations to the natural world and how are we responsible for enabling other humans and other creatures in their relationship to nature? These questions are appropriate to mystery, in this case the mystery of the natural world—despite our enormous amount of knowledge about it, it remains a challenge we will never exhaust, provoking us to reflect hard and long about the meaning of human life in this world.

The example from cognitive science proceeds similarly. The more we learn about our brains and how their processes correlate to our mental lives, the deeper the mystery of how our neurobiology can enable the unbelievably rich possibilities that our minds explore every moment, whether it is creative art, problem-solving, devising strategies for living, or deepening our relationships with other people. In these activities, our minds—in their thoroughly natural biological working—do in fact continuously transcend our physical situations. In this mental activity, nature is transcending itself. We would put a different spin on Katherine Hepburn's line about nature as that which we must rise above—nature is always rising above itself, because it is a continuously self-transcending realm. When we ponder the meaning of human life in the natural world and when we experience the creativity of Shakespeare or the inventor, author, and Google's chief of engineering Ray Kurzweil we experience nature itself seeking to go beyond itself. Our encounter with mystery is a signal that we are in the presence of transcendence that challenges us to explore its depths.

---

9. Sutera, *Work of God*, 81.

We think of Teilhard's aphorism, "Humans are evolution aware of itself."[10] In our very own intellectual and spiritual life, we witness nature going beyond itself, and we embody this witness in our experience; it is ours—*the witness is us*, if you will. While we possess this self-transcending action, since it is our own experience, at the same time we are aware that we are not fully in control of its cascading rush; we sense that we are riding a torrent that is larger than we are—we are subject and object at the same time. Rather than possessing this experience, it is more accurate to say that we are possessed in it. Here we are confronted with the basic question: What is the significance of these acts of transcendence? What do they reveal to us about our fundamental human nature and our reason for being? Again we encounter, not a lack of knowledge, not a puzzle to be resolved, but the mystery of our very bodily nature—this is Tillich's point: our nature possesses a mystery, a depth, and a greatness that are fully natural.

(6) *Full-bodied/God-intoxicated*. These reflections lead to a sixth idea of nature: *Full-bodied/God-intoxicated*. We call this idea—that nature is the inexhaustible source from which new things continually emerge—a *full-bodied* idea of nature. As such, nature continually confronts us with and wraps us in *mystery*. Mystery involves us, as we have said, in transcendence, and when religious people encounter transcendence and mystery, they understand that they are in the presence of God. We must be clear—this engagement with transcendence and God comes to us, *not* through some supernatural intervention and not by introducing some *unnatural* element. Rather, we are through earthiness bathed in transcendence. Hence, we call this a *full-bodied* and *God-intoxicated* idea of nature.

These ideas of nature, particularly nature as a process of emergence and as full-bodied/God-intoxicated, bring with them a deep sense of humility. We are very much aware of ourselves as being borne upon processes of which we are not the authors or the drivers. We know ourselves to be in possession of freedom, in that we are always faced with decisions that need to be made. Even more, we feel that we are part of something bigger than ourselves, and this is the seed of humility in the face of nature—both within us and outside of us. This sense of humility in the face of depth has been called "creature-feeling"; we engage mystery at this point. Mystery surrounds us at every point: when we seek knowledge of nature, when we try to control it, when we ponder its bottomless depth within us—each of these is an avenue that leads us sooner or later to mystery, which in turn

10. Teihard de Chardin, *The Phenomenon of Man*, 220.

is an opening to transcendence. The poet A. R. Ammons spoke of how "things spiral out from a center" and take shape as they come forth.[11] The processes of nature on which we are borne are always spiraling out from mystery and taking shape right before us—and within us.

A CHRISTIAN IDEA OF NATURE

Recall at the beginning of this chapter, we noted Collingwood's point that our idea of nature touches upon everything else we believe. If we hold to the idea that nature is analogous to a machine, for example, we cannot include emergence as a natural occurrence, because emergence does not happen in machines; the machine is what it is because of its maker or mechanic, and the maker is outside the machine. We could not consider ourselves to be fully natural, because we are, fundamentally, not machines, nor could we think of God in nature, since God is not machine-like. If we follow the analogy of nature as living organism, we could not include quantum subatomic physics in nature, nor molecular and nano-levels, because they are not living organisms. We would also have to endorse a version of Intelligent Design theory—that nature possesses an intelligent mind. According to these analogies, God must be "up there," and "out there" in some realm that is not "nature," or "back there" as a First Cause, because God is neither machine nor organism. Further these analogies do not allow us to view ourselves as fully natural creatures. By today's standards, these ideas of nature are anti-science.

For us, nature is best understood *as historical process of emergence that continually brings us face-to-face with mystery—full-bodied and God intoxicated*—precisely because these analogies allow us to see ourselves as fully natural and God's presence as fully capable of expressing itself within nature.

Now we are in a position to understand nature in a Christian sense. Let me recap some features of this idea of nature:

1. It is not a scientific idea of nature, but rather a philosophical/theological interpretation of nature taking into account both scientific knowledge and our common experience. It is consistent with science, since it does not contradict scientific findings. It goes beyond science, but not against science. Science does not in itself affirm God, but as it

11. Ammons, "Poetics," 199, lines 2–3.

unfolds nature for us, it brings us to the point where God is a viable interpretation of our experience of nature.

2. On the contrary, I emphasize how science has so totally expanded our view of nature, compelling us to work within the parameters of the "turn to nature" that I described at the outset and at the same time revealing that nature is both the all-encompassing ambience for our lives, and also the self-transcending energy that points us to mystery and ultimacy.

3. This idea of nature does not engage in "God of the gaps" strategies. I am not seizing upon any inadequacy of science in order to make a theological point. I bring mystery into the discussion, with science actually an agent of that mystery. It is when we take with utter seriousness the advances in scientific knowledge that we are brought up against mystery—as I try to show in my examples from climate change and cognitive neuroscience. There is no point in hoping to find God in some supposed gaps or inadequacies in scientific knowledge.

4. It is not necessary in light of this idea of nature to bring God into the discussion, but intelligent people can agree that God is certainly a possibility. One thing I do insist on: that we acknowledge that science itself brings us into situations where questions arise, choices must be made that cannot be resolved by scientific reasoning. Science itself brings to the point where we must go beyond science in some way in order to deal with our scientific knowledge.

Collingwood believed that our idea of nature conditions what we believe about everything else. It is like a backboard off which we bounce our ideas about other things. What does the full-bodied/God-intoxicated idea of nature suggest about how we view humans and ourselves? (1) That our lives, including their mental and spiritual dimensions run their course as processes of nature, even though they defy naturalistic reductionism. Our minds and spirits are not unnatural add-ons, nor are they outside nature. (2) We are nature, as much as anything in this world, and as such everything we say about nature transpires within us and our lives—whether as described by physics, biology, chemistry, neuroscience, or any other science—including the social and historical sciences. (3) Nature that is us is as fully described by knowledge, control, and mystery as any other natural phenomena—indeed even more so.

What does the idea of nature that I have presented suggest about God? (1) That nature is a God-friendly domain—which we would expect since God created it out of nothing and is the sole source of nature. (2) God inhabits nature and lives in, with, and under natural processes and phenomena. In the next section, we bring in the Christian theological witness to this divine presence in nature. The witnesses are deeply ensconced in the tradition—in the affirmations of the incarnation, the two natures of Christ, and the traditions of the communication of attributes (*communicatio idiomatum*) between the divine and the human in Christ, and in our sacramental traditions.

CHRISTIAN BELIEF IN CHRIST AS INTERPRETATION OF NATURE

We are now in a position to explore some very rich elements of the Christian tradition. We begin with the classic symbol of the incarnation. Incarnation is the specifically Christian way of referring to God's dwelling in the world in Jesus of Nazareth. It is symbolic and dogmatic shorthand for the saying in Revelation 21:3: "See, the home of God is among mortals. He will dwell with them as their God." The Gospel of John puts this more abstractly in the first chapter: "In the beginning was the Word, and the Word was with God, and the Word was God. . . . [A]ll things were made through him, and without him was not anything made that was made. . . . And the Word became flesh and dwelt among us" (KJV).

What we have here grows out of the intuitive responses of early Christians to the impact that this man Jesus made upon them. Very soon, however, the intuitions became subjects of reflection, and that continues to the present time. How is it possible for God to dwell among us, to become material flesh? Affirming incarnation is to affirm something about nature as a whole and about our own human nature. As the Franciscan theologian Zachary Hayes has said, to assert incarnation brings God into play with physics, biology, and all the rest of what we know about nature.[12]

The process of reflection on what the basic Christian assertion means for nature began very early and its shape is imprinted in a number of historical markers. We will focus on several of these: the Council of Chalcedon's formulation of the so-called "two natures" of Christ and Leo's Tome, from the fifth century; the medieval maxim that "grace does not destroy nature,

---

12. Hayes, *A Window to the Divine*.

but presupposes and undergirds it"; and the sixteenth- and seventeenth-century argumentation about the "communication of attributes" between Christ's human and divine natures. The last two items are not covered here. There is no intention of offering a detailed and comprehensive discussion of Christian tradition. Rather, in line with our method of scenes or snapshots and vignettes, we dip into the tradition to retrieve certain key episodes to form our picture of a self-transcending natural body—and eventually our idea of ourselves as God's bodyselves.

CHALCEDON AND LEO—JESUS CHRIST'S BODY ON THE CUSP OF TRANSCENDENCE

When we read the original documents of faith that were formed in the middle of the fifth century, we appreciate the passion and the freshness with which they wrestle with the human nature they knew in Jesus. Even though we speak of the chronologically late-in-the-day idea of nature I proposed previously in this chapter (a process of emergence and as full-bodied/God-intoxicated), eras earlier than ours experienced nature in a similar way, but strained to give expression to their experience. Their Christian sensibility could not be contained in the prevailing philosophy and language of their time. The Hellenistic culture in which Christianity was born had neither the dictionary of words nor the glossary of philosophical concepts to interpret their experience adequately. Scientific knowledge today is in fact liberating their experience from the limitations of their thought-world. Perhaps for the first time, Christian belief in the incarnation finds itself set in a worldview that enables fuller expression of this belief and its implications—and it is science that has enabled this new situation, with a new dictionary and a new glossary of concepts, to emerge. We are witnessing the excitement of discovery that an ancient traditional formulation can actually give expression to a contemporary breakthrough in our understanding of nature. We affirm the truth of Paul Ricoeur's insight that words are never imprisoned in the expressions of a single author or a single age—they break out with explosive force—they reveal possibilities of meaning that cannot be suppressed or be strait-jacketed by any single interpretation.[13] Words and images can in fact mean whatever they are capable of meaning.

Let us focus on some passages from Leo (448 CE) and from the Council of Chalcedon's formulation (451 CE) to make this point. The subject of

13. Ricoeur, *The Rule of Metaphor*.

discussion, we recall, is the nature of Jesus Christ—that he is both divine and human. Leo states:

> While the distinctness of both natures and substances is preserved, and both meet in one Person, lowliness is assumed by majesty, weakness by power, mortality by eternity . . . the man Christ Jesus might from one element be capable of dying and from the other be incapable. Therefore in the entire and perfect nature of very man was born very God, whole in what was his, whole in what was ours. It is equally dangerous to believe the Lord Jesus Christ to be merely God and not man or merely man and not God.[14]

The critical point here is that in the incarnation human nature and divinity each retains its integrity—distinct and uncompromised, while at the same time they are indissolubly united in one whole human person. There is no talk of "half human/half divine" or some mixture; Jesus is no Minotaur nor is the divinity dissolved in the humanity like sugar in a cup of tea. This is what the dogma means to say: oneness in unity, humanity and divinity—both uncompromised. The terminology by which historians and theologians identify the dogma—"two natures in one person"—is itself inadequate for us today, since its intent is to affirm a *oneness* in the face of twoness and not a dualism between the human and the divine.

The Chalcedonian Formulation makes the same affirmation, if anything, more emphatically, in both simple, "truly God and truly man," and technical, "like unto God in his divinity, like unto us in his humanity," language. Then follow the famous four "without's": "*without* confusion, *without* change, *without* division, *without* separation" (in the original Greek, the celebrated four "alpha privatives").[15] The first two rule out intermingling and watering down—we're dealing with real humanity and real divinity. The second pair preserves the unity—Jesus was not a split personality, not a split person.

These two foundational documents—the heart of the dogma of the so-called two natures—take some thinking about, they are not easy to digest. They are difficult, because they obviously do not make sense; they are counterintuitive; they demand that we think new thoughts—that we open ourselves to a new worldview, in Collingwood's jargon, a new idea of nature.

---

14. Leo the Great, "The Tome of Leo," 363.
15. Council of Chalcedon, "Chalcedonian Decree," 373.

Christian faith and theology carried the thread of this classic idea of nature forward into the Middle Ages in a powerful way. It never abandoned the belief that nature is the earthen vessel of God's presence and grace. Theologians elaborated this in the much quoted aphorism: "grace *presupposes* nature; it does not destroy it, but rather conserves and perfects it"; the original Latin can also be translated as: "grace *undergirds* nature; it does not destroy it, but rather conserves and perfects it."

Christian faith is frequently depicted as being unfriendly to nature—an embodiment of the Katherine Hepburn view. This strand of ideas stemming from Chalcedon and continuing through the Middle Ages has never dropped out of the faith tradition. This fact takes on all the more importance when we consider how difficult it is to hold this interpretation of nature in the face of the naturalistic and materialistic views that assume nature is a one-dimensional realm. Protestant theologians in the sixteenth and seventeenth centuries present some of the clearest examples of how belief in the God-intoxicated idea of nature can appear both dogged and tortured. Focusing on how the "attributes" of humanity and divinity could coexist within the human body of Jesus, they sometimes associated each with specific human properties. For example, Lutheran theologian Martin Chemnitz argues while the divine nature of Christ could not suffer, it was active in permitting the human nature to do, while in performing miracles, the human nature allows itself to be stretched by the divine nature beyond its finite limits.[16] Even though the attempted precision of the analysis may seem to us today as enormous scholastic baggage, it stands as testimony to the seriousness with which these thinkers took the vision of the incarnation.

How God relates to the created, material world is a mystery. After all, God does not exist in the same way that things exist in this world; God is infinite, in contrast to the finitude that we live in. From this angle, God and the world of nature appear to be quite separate—even "other."

The nineteenth-century thinker, Søren Kierkegaard, spoke of the infinite qualitative difference between God and the world—a coinage that affirms the fourth-century formulation we mentioned earlier, *apophatic*.[17] That earlier concept emphasizes that the majesty and mystery of God so far transcend our human minds that in our attempts to know God we are speechless, bereft of words and concepts that can grasp the Infinite. Without

---

16. Chemnitz, *De duabus naturis in Christo* 27, cited in Schmid, *Doctrinal Theology*, 343–4.

17. Kierkegaard, *Concluding Unscientific Postscript*, esp. 186–98.

weakening our awareness of this infinite qualitative difference, Christian faith nevertheless holds that God's presence is one of grace and that it undergirds the natural world and our natural bodies and works to conserve and perfect them. Kierkegaard called this a "paradox."[18] Nature and our bodies do not appear to be undergirded by grace and transcendence, but in Christian perspective, they are.

So what? Why is this important? Because it provides a point of contact with our contemporary view of ourselves as creatures of nature, and because it allows us to accept and understand our experience and knowledge of nature as opening out to mystery. Further, it points us to the significance of that mystery—it is the face of ultimacy, the very ground of the natural world; in other words, nature opens us to God. We come face-to-face with a two-sided reality: (1) Once-and-for-all we must recognize that nature is not a one-dimensional domain upon which we can perform a reductionism of any sort, or which we can fully know or control. In this, the dogmas disclose to us a deep truth about our science and our technology. *They entail a paradox: they float on the surface of reality that is much deeper and more mysterious than they know, even as at the same time, in their quest for knowledge and control, they in fact open up that depth and mystery.* (2) At the same time, we are compelled to see that what we consider to be ultimate or transcendent or divine—however we think of God or the most really real—is in, with, and under what we experience as nature. God is not "out there," but rather *in there,* deeper and more constitutive than we can imagine. God doesn't *need to be* "out there." Nature never ceases to be earthy, fully natural, fully big-bang stardust, fully embedded in the thermodynamic processes of evolution, fully biochemical, fully neurobiological—it is not changed. Nature is fully itself, *distinct and uncompromised,* as the ancient formulation insists. But God, transcendent depth, is indissolubly united with this nature, equally distinct and uncompromised.

Gerard Manley Hopkins attempted with some success to express this radical view of nature in his 1877 poem, "God's Grandeur," when he wrote that "The world is charged with the grandeur of God. . . . nature is never spent; / there lives the dearest freshness deep down things."[19] Fully natural yet somehow *charged* with genuine transcendence—deep down things, deeper than we can ever go.

---

18. Kierkegaard, *Philosophical Fragments,* 46–67.
19. Hopkins, "God's Grandeur," 66; also Hopkins, "God's Grandeur," online edition.

Here we come upon another facet of our experience of nature—our intuitive sense of the freshness deep down things. This intuition is embodied in another traditional Christian expression—sacramental life. When Christians share the Holy Communion or Eucharist or Mass, they enter a world rich with symbols and myths that speak of the nature of nature that we have been reflecting on. They hold bread, common ordinary bread, in their hands and they drink ordinary wine. They hear the words, "This bread is my body broken for you, this wine is my blood poured out for you." We are reminded that in the original Aramaic that Jesus spoke, the word "is" did not occur—the first participants heard only "bread/body, wine/blood." We consume the bread/body and wine/blood, and they undergo one of the earthiest, most natural processes imaginable—digestion and metabolism. Bread and wine become bone of our bone and flesh of our flesh. Moreover, Christians call this union with God. This is "sacrament," referred to in earliest times as *mystery (musterion)*. How could natural things share in this highly symbolic transaction? An expansive idea of nature is required even to imagine it.

The larger symbolic meaning here is that each of us is a sacrament, in an earthy human body living on the cusp of transcendence. Further, that the entire world is sacramental mystery. Teilhard de Chardin's *Mass on the World* was conceived when he was on the arduous Yellow Expedition across China's Gobi desert in the late 1920s.[20] The *Mass* portrays exactly this, that the planet is Christ's body and that by living in this world, one participates in sacramental reality. Citing Gregory of Nyssa (fourth century), he writes, "The bread of the Eucharist is stronger than our flesh; that is why it is the bread that assimilates us, and not we the bread, when we receive it."[21] The bread, which is the body of Christ, consumes us. Teilhard was a mystic, and he writes in that vein in elaborating this view:

> Since Christ is above all omega, that is, the universal "form" of the world, he can attain his organic balance and plenitude only by mystically assimilating all that surrounds him. The Host is like a blazing hearth from which flames spread their radiance. Just as the spark that falls into the heather is soon surrounded by a wide circle of fire, so the sacramental Host of bread is continually being

---

20. Teihard de Chardin, "The Mass on the World," 9–33.
21. Teilhard de Chardin, "My Universe," 65.

encircled more closely by another, infinitely larger, Host, which is nothing less than the universe itself.[22]

The worshippers sharing in this ritual are far from possessing a full-blown intellectual comprehension of what they are doing and praying. Nevertheless, within the ambience of the images and the ritual actions, they intuit deeper possibilities for nature—the natural bread and wine, their own bodily lives, the world, and the universe—transcendent possibilities. The Lutheran tradition of which I am part affirms that precise philosophical language cannot take the measure of this sacramental experience, hence their non-technical language, that the transcendence is "in, with, and under" the natural forms. The intuition here is one of deeper meaning, but it also an intuition of *hope*—hope for what this experience can disclose, hope for what nature is and can become. Hope for what the persons and their world can become.

It is a simple matter to classify what I have described here as ancient tradition, as particularistic ritual, as a premodern worldview. As such, our task is to overcome it—that is what the Enlightenment proposed. I am suggesting, however, that this tradition is also an interpretation of nature. Furthermore, that it is an interpretation of nature as understood by contemporary science. Even more, I am arguing that nothing less than this or some comparable explanation can take the measure of what we know about nature through science and how we experience it.

We require such a new, expansive idea of nature if we hope to comprehend our own amazing nature—our bodyselves.

---

22. Ibid., 65; also, Hefner, "Teilhard's Spiritual Vision," 79–94.

10

Luther on the Body
Incarnation, Sacrament, Technoself, and Faith

Ann Milliken Pederson

WE KNOW THAT OUR identity emerges from the entangled and extended relationships in which our bodyselves are embedded. We are technobody selves, tethered in, with, and under the technologies and social media that create our personhood. Many of us embody multiple identities and selves: virtual, real, male, female, inter-sex, poor, rich, middle-class, young, older, dying, birthing, viable, fetus, embryo, child, and adult. We will resist being explained by "nothing buts" and simplistic labels. We can celebrate the multidimensional nature of our bodyselves, whose relationship to the world, both past and into the future, emerges through entangled and extended webs of otherness. This is the flesh of incarnation, flesh into which God is also embedded and extended. The Christian tradition and Scriptures relate narratives about this creation and God who is incarnate in the world. Christians have used sacramental language to convey this: God present is in, with, and under the finite elements of this world. So what does this mean in light of medicine, healthcare, and biotechnology?

Martin Luther's theological views on the human body and body of Christ are complicated. He addresses embodiment at several levels: the physical/material incarnation of Jesus as divine/human (Chalcedonian understanding), the body of Christ in the Eucharist, the body of Christ as church, the institutional bodies in power, and the human condition as faith in an embodied spirit. What ties them all together? The way that faith becomes embodied in lived experience.

Luther doesn't shy away from very earthy, physical descriptions of his faith and his theology: his supposed conversion whilst in the bathroom, throwing inkwells at the devil, singing hymns, and playing the lute, denying his body through practices in his early life as a monk and later being troubled by hemorrhoids, and the vivid images of intimacy and earthliness he uses to describe the believer's relationship to God in Christ. Margaret Miles, church historian and theologian, notes: "Luther's references to present embodied experience range widely, as is well known, from the trivialization of the body in some of his scatological remarks to profoundly loving statements about the care of the body as a 'Christian work.'"[1] In his dialectical use of flesh and spirit, Luther describes "flesh" as the whole person who is oriented away from God and "spirit" as the bodyself's orientation towards God. What made the Reformation so powerful was the physical embodiment of the Reformers' ideas. Luther literally re-embodied the practices of his understanding of the Christian faith, which in turn change the "minds" of the believers.

What interests me more now than ever as I think is how radically embodied we are, that concepts like the "mind of Christ" are about the extended embodiment of God in the world. Luther's theology was radical because it changed not only people's "minds," but also their bodies. The Reformation, in a sense, was a full-scale challenge to previous embodiments of the Christian faith at that time. Some of the radical embodiments of Luther's notion of faith came from physical acts. Here are some of his ideas and how they embody the Christian gospel.

Luther created a distinction between flesh and spirit, and yet it was one that did not denigrate flesh. "Nor does Paul demand of the faithful that they completely destroy and kill the flesh, but that they control it in such a way that it will be subject to the Spirit."[2] The spirit must control the flesh. We satisfy our needs and not our desires. One should even take care of their bodies. "For just as we should not be cruel to other people's bodies or trouble them with unjust requirements, so we should not do this to our own bodies either."[3]

---

1. Miles, "The Rope Breaks," 253.
2. *LW* 27:69.
3. Ibid.

The Spirit can free us from the terrors we experience that seem to be from the flesh. The Spirit can heal us by knowing that these terrors are beyond our control. "It often happens that a man is so fiercely attacked by anger, hatred, impatience, sexual desire, mental depression, or some other desire of the flesh that he simply cannot get rid of it, no matter how much he wants to. What is he to do? Should he despair on this account?"[4] While I'm not making Luther out to be some kind of psychotherapist, he clearly understands that experiences like depression or anxiety can be beyond human control and that it is not a sign of "being condemned." The Spirit frees the whole person, and God's grace heals us from the effects of the flesh. "Therefore God stretches the immense heaven of grace over us and for the sake of Christ does not impute to us the remnants of sin that cling to our flesh."[5] The flesh applies to our entire being.

The experience of faith is not just an interior feeling but it involves the whole bodyself. "Therefore one's spirit must be trained, so that when it becomes conscious of the accusation of the Law, the terrors of sin, the horror of death, and wrath of God, it will banish these sorrowful scenes from its sight and will replace them with the freedom of Christ, the forgiveness of sins, righteousness, life, and the eternal mercy of God."[6] This practice or training of the spirit is in contrast to the practice or training that Luther experienced in the monastery. For Luther, the monastic practices led to a kind of physical-spiritual anxiety, like theological panic attacks. But to practice the faith or train one's life in the Spirit of Christ can lead to joy and trust in God. "The comfort is this, that in your deep anxieties—in which your consciousness of sin, sadness, and despair is so great and strong that it penetrates and occupies all the corners of your heart—you do not follow your consciousness."[7] Luther said we follow the Word of God that leads us to mercy and the tenderhearted nature of God.

The language of Luther on the experience of the law and of the gospel is replete with physical language. This was not simply an "intellectually abstract" doctrine, but was felt deeply within the body of the believer. Faith is not simple passivity, but activity through the Spirit. "Therefore Christians are really runners; whatever they do runs along and moves forward successfully, being advanced by the Spirit of Christ, who has nothing to do

---

4. *LW* 27:78.
5. *LW* 27:86.
6. *LW* 27:5.
7. *LW* 27:26.

with slow enterprises."[8] Thus the experience of faith involves not only the body of the believer, but also the bodies of the neighbor, especially those who suffer and are in need. When one is faithful in their Christian life, the body of Christ becomes manifest. "As I have said, therefore, Paul is describing the whole of the Christian life in this passage: inwardly it is faith toward God, and outwardly it is love or works toward one's neighbor."[9] For Luther, the neighbor was the one in need, the lowly. "For your brother does not stop being your neighbor simply because he lapses or because he offends you, but that is the very time when he needs your love for him the most."[10] To love and serve the neighbor is the embodiment of faith.

Luther inverts the body of Christ from the way he saw the Romanists vision of the body of God by developing his notion of the priesthood of all believers.[11] In his "Treatise to the German Nobility," Luther links power and embodiment. "We must not start something by trusting in great power or human reason, even if all the power in the world were ours. For God cannot and will not suffer that a good work begins by relying on one's own power and reason."[12] What people needed was a church who are a community of believers who take care of the neighbor and empower each other for good. The body of Christ becomes the body through the power of Christ and not from the spiritual powers of the papacy. "All Christians are truly of the spiritual estate, and there is no difference among them except that of office."[13] Christians are all members of one body, yet every member serves the one body in different ways.

Luther embodied the gospel in the way he understood the architecture of the sanctuary and in the way he celebrated the Eucharist. For example, he gave communion in both kinds. Kurt Hendel, a Lutheran Reformation historian and theologian writes: "In light of the doctrine of the priesthood of all believers and his insistence that the sacrament was Christ's gift to the whole community, not a passion of the clergy, Luther also advocated that the altar should be moved away from the wall and that the priest should

---

8. *LW* 27:32.

9. *LW* 27:30.

10. *LW* 27:65.

11. Luther challenges the three walls of the Romanists who claim that spiritual power does not have power above the temporal, that only the Pope can interpret Scripture, and that only the Pope may summon a council.

12. Luther, "Treatise to the German Nobility," 9.

13. Ibid., 12.

face the people during the sacramental liturgy."[14] When the celebrant faced the congregation, this physical act of turning toward embodied the relationship of the congregation to God through the sacraments.

Luther's support of music and the visual arts were ways to hear and see the Word of God. His translations of the Bible into the vernacular also included many woodcuts, some even in color.[15] These acts brought the gospel to life through the bodily senses so Christians could experience the gospel in multiple ways.

I think that one of the reasons that the Reformation spread so quickly is that Luther not only challenged the doctrine and ideas of the Papacy, but also, and maybe most importantly, the embodiments and practices of the Christian faith. Luther's way of doing theology does not involve speculation on abstract ideas, but involves becoming completely immersed in the world's problems: "It is by living—no rather, by dying and being damned that a theologian is made, not by understanding, reading or speculating."[16] For Luther, theological knowledge is always embodied and it is "not a matter of speculation either, but completely of practice and feeling."[17] Several centuries later, Dietrich Bonhoeffer, shared that same vision of faith: "In Christ, we are invited to participate in the reality of God and the reality of the world at the same time, the one not without the other. The reality of God is disclosed only as it places me completely into the reality of the world."[18] For Luther, the incarnation of God in the world and in the person of Jesus the Christ has to do with salvation—that is, to do for creation what we cannot do. The incarnate and human God is the God who creates and redeems the world.[19] For Luther, as well as for others, salvation is not just about a personal relationship with Jesus Christ, but also begins from and must include the healing of and reconciliation of all creation—that all shall be well. This incarnational emphasis comes to full expression in his soteriological and sacramental metaphor of the joyous or happy exchange.

Luther's image of the "joyous exchange" dramatizes how intimate and embodied the relationship between Christ and the believer is and this is

14. Hendel, "*Finitum capax infiniti*," 431.

15. Ibid.

16. Luther, ". . . *vivendo, immo moriendo et damnando fit theologus, non itelligendo, legend aut speculando*," WA, 163.

17. Luther, *LW*, 12, 311.

18. Bonhoeffer, *Ethics*, 55.

19. Luther, *LW* 26:28.

experienced in particular for the Christian through the sacraments. The sacraments are tangible proof of God's promises because they come through the bodyself in which we receive them. Unlike the Sacramentarians, with whom Luther argues at length, who claim that the finite is not capable of bearing the infinite, Luther claims that the tangible, physical presence of Christ is precisely *where* God promises to be present for us. But God is not only incarnate in the faith of the believer, but also in the entirety of the creation. Luther claimed that all of creation is good and that God is intimately present in all of creation, not just human bodies. Christ's flesh is a soteriological issue for Luther: nothing is beyond the scope of God's grace. The finite world, for Luther, was not one part of a dualism between the finite and the infinite. *Finitum capax infiniti*—in a manger, in the leaves on a tree, in human bodyselves—there God is present for us.

Luther uses intimate physical language in both metaphorical and literal ways to describe where God is present in the creation. Luther writes: "Indeed, he makes and does nothing except through his Word, Genesis 1 and John 1, i.e. his power. Then if his power and Spirit are present everywhere and in all things to the innermost and outermost degree, through and through, as it must be if he is to take and preserve all things everywhere, then his right hand, nature, majesty, must also be everywhere. He must be present if he makes and preserves them."[20]

One can see Luther opening the way for what today is called panentheistic theology—God is both distinct from, but also intimately involved in the world. The world is seen as God's body—the creation (humanity included) is God's body. Luther writes that God is located "in, and through the whole creation in all of its parts and in all places, and so the world is full of God and he fills it all . . . ."[21] This language is helpful because it avoids a dualism in which a giant abyss separates God and the world that only Jesus the Christ can bridge. Instead, Luther speaks of this intimate presence of God that has "found the way whereby his own divine nature can be wholly and entirely in all creatures and in every single being, more deeply, more inwardly, more present that the creature is to itself . . . ."[22] It is not a stretch to claim that Luther leads to the notion the world is to God like a baby is in the womb of its mother.

20. *LW,* 37:61.
21. *LW* 37:59.
22. *LW* 37:60.

Because God became incarnate in Christ and Christ is in us, we can experience the joy and pleasure of our bodyselves, gifts from our creator God. Luther would, of course, have read the early church fathers—Irenaeus, Athanasius, the Cappadocians. Their understanding of faith, which is later developed into the language of the Orthodox notion of *theosis*, summarizes this process of becoming the bodyself that God calls us to be. In *The Bondage of the Will*, Luther writes that "here John says that believers are born of God and become the children of God—become, indeed, gods, new creatures."[23] The one who has faith becomes divine, and of course, for Luther, like the author of Philippians, divinity was best understood as taking on the flesh of the lowest position in society. Luther: "The one who has faith is a completely divine man, a son of God, the inheritor of the universe."[24] We become divine so that we can take on the needs of our neighbor. Embodiment comes in a crucified form—to be the body of Christ for the neighbor. The Christian faith is always connected to the needs of the neighbor:

> yet God does not work in us without us; for He created and preserves us for this very purpose, that He might work in us and we might cooperate with Him, whether that occurs outside His kingdom, by His general omnipotence, or within His kingdom, by the special power of the Holy Spirit . . . . For He creates and preserves us for this very purpose that He might work in us and we might cooperate with Him. Thus he preaches, shows mercy to the poor, and comforts the afflicted by means of us.[25]

To be a bodyself is to be in relationship to God and the neighbor, in particular those who are suffering. God becomes incarnate within us so that we might become incarnate in others. Christians, like Christ, are called to enter into that which is not so "pleasing" or lovely to the world so that those bodyselves who feel devalued and unpleasing can know that they are vital and pleasing to God and to others. The incarnation can be a vehicle of affirmation for the human person—that we are good and loved, not for what we do or what parts of our body we can sell or have used by others—we are simply loved.

---

23. Luther, *Bondage of the Will*, 269.
24. *LW*, 26:247.
25. Luther, *Bondage of the Will*, 268.

11

The Body of Christ

Ann Milliken Pederson

I'VE ALWAYS WANTED TO be a part of the body of Christ, but the body of Christ has not always wanted me in it. I grew up in the Lutheran church: attending Sunday school, singing in the choir, and going to camp in the summer. In junior high school, when someone asked me what I wanted to do when I grew up, I could answer: I want to be a pastor. The church, however, did not always inspire my love of the church. In confirmation, our pastor told us to sit in every other seat and we were rarely allowed to ask questions. For two years, we endured his lectures at us. I remember talking with my mother about wanting to quit. The only reason to continue was that in order to commune I had to be confirmed. I still remember the white robes we wore as we marched into the sanctuary and took our first communion. Most of us were around thirteen years old. In high school I listened to Bach, learned more about the life of Martin Luther, and read some of the existential philosophers in my literature classes. Thinking about theological questions came naturally to me and I loved the musical traditions of the Reformers. This was the part of the church that I loved and in which I felt at home. But that was not my only experience of being Lutheran or being a part of the church.

My home church in Montana was caught in the very same conflicts of the culture of its times—women were demanding gender equality, African Americans marched with dignity for civil rights, and the churches were struggling to hold on to traditions that once held them together while at the same time trying to also address the newer and often younger voices that challenged those very traditions. When I first thought about attending seminary, I heard from my pastor and youth pastor that women should not be ordained. They told me that simply because I was female I could not be a part of the body of Christ in the way that I felt called to be. For the first time in my life, I was told that my body didn't fit into the body of Christ. I was angry and didn't understand that the very church that I loved and wanted to be a part of would reject me because of my femaleness. It wasn't long into my last year of junior high school that the exclusion of women from ordained ministry was challenged and change happened. In 1970 in the Lutheran Church, women were ordained into ministry. In 1979 I entered Luther Seminary in St. Paul, Minnesota. Approximately 10 percent of the entering seminary class was women. Now, those numbers have changed drastically. Women comprise at least half of most entering seminary classes in the Evangelical Lutheran Church in American (ELCA). The body of Christ does indeed change.

However, while the ELCA now includes women, other denominations still exclude women from ordained ministry, often quoting the same sources and giving the same reasons that I heard decades ago: Jesus was male and so were all his disciples. Other church authorities quote the deuteropauline and Pauline Epistles or make arguments using a form of natural law—all used to exclude women from the body of Christ.[1] Women have been and still are excluded as full partners in the body of Christ. But so are people who are gay and lesbian, bisexual and transgender. So are the poor and those people whose bodies are disabled. What has become clear to me is that the body of Christ never has been and never will be some perfect entity because it is made up of the bodies of finite, flawed humans. From the very beginning of its origins, the body of Christ, which is called church, reflects the bodies of those who are both in its boundaries and of those who have been excluded from it. Paul's letters to the various communities with whom he ministered reflect these same struggles. In each generation, problems

1. Deuteropauline epistles: New Testament letters attributed to Paul, but which, in the view of most biblical scholars, are not: i.e., 2 Thessalonians, Colossians, Ephesians, 1–2 Timothy, and Titus. The Pauline Epistles: The New Testament letters considered by most scholars to be written or dictated by Paul.

about the diversity and the unity of the church arise and each generation confronts them in their own way. Simply put: because Christianity is an incarnational faith, the body of Christ, the church, reflects the experiences of the human bodies of which it is comprised. And like Paul and all of those who came with and after him, the church struggles to figure out what that means. And that struggle is especially important in light of those who the church continues to exclude, or whose bodily experience is discounted or marginalized.

What does it mean for Christians today to be part of the body of Christ? We cannot give a simple response to that question. We do know that human bodyselves are extremely complex, diverse, and profoundly different from one another. Like Paul and those who came after him, we struggle with the metaphor of what it means to be the body of Christ. Rather than abandon that language, we hope we can expand and enrich it. We need new metaphors for what it means to be church in the twenty-first century because we are seeking a more complex, deeper understanding of what it means to be human. We claim that the body of Christ is not in some other invisible place, in some mystical realm apart from the messiness of our daily lives, but indeed, the body of Christ is us—we *are* church. To draw clean lines between some mystical or invisible body of Christ and the church as institution seems ambiguous at best, and false at the worst. The church as body of Christ lives out the tensions of the individuals within it and the structures of the institutions that sustain and order it. The church bears the tension of what is now and what is not yet—the ways in which Christ is present now and in ways that are yet to be. Instead of prescribing what the church should be, we offer some stories and descriptions of ways it might be and maybe already is. We hope these images and stories will draw us into participating more fully in the body of Christ and into more complex and healing relationships with the creation around us. Instead of excluding and drawing lines that separate and divide, we should err on the side of including and unifying. In a world in which religion turns "us" into "them," and friends into enemies, we hope that the body of Christ is not merely a metaphor, but a reality of God's grace that heals divisions, offers compassion to those who suffer, and provides dignity for those who have been deemed worthless. Where do we start our theological task? Where Scripture itself starts . . . in the garden.

THE MESSY GARDEN

The following quotes from Donna Haraway, a scholar of science and technology, and from the Bible, link our beginnings in nature to our understanding of who we are as bodyselves. All the quotes capture the messiness and complexity of gardens. When God created the world, God pronounced it good, but not perfect!

Haraway writes: "And like the productions of a decadent gardener who can't keep the good distinctions between natures and cultures straight, my shape of my kin networks looks more like a trellis or an esplanade than a tree. You can't tell up from down, and everything seems to go sidewise. Such snake-like, sidewinding traffic is one of my themes. My garden is full of snakes, full of trellises, full of indirection."[2]

> And the Lord God planted a garden in Eden, in the east; and there he put the man whom he had formed. Out of the ground the Lord God made to grow every tree that is pleasant to the sight and good for food, the tree of life also in the midst of the garden, and the tree of the knowledge of good and evil. (Gen 2:4b, 8–9)
>
> They heard the sound of the Lord God walking in the garden at the time of the evening breeze, and the man and his wife hid themselves from the presence of the Lord God among the trees of the garden. (Gen 3:8)
>
> My beloved speaks and says to me: "Arise, my love, my fair one, and come away; for now the winter is past, the rain is over and gone. The flowers appear on the earth; the time of singing has come, and the voice of the turtledove is heard in our land. The fig tree puts forth its figs, and the vines are in blossom; they give forth fragrance. (Song 2:10, 13)
>
> He is the image of the invisible God, the firstborn of all creation; for in him all things in heaven and on earth were created, things visible and invisible, whether thrones or dominions or rulers or powers—all things have been created through him and for him. He himself is before all things, and in him all things hold together. (Col 1:15–17)

What we need is a vision of the church that can mold and inform a new, imaginative, and provocative way of helping us to interpret our vocation and place within the universe. What is our vocation and place within God's creation? To answer that question, we will begin where Scripture does: within the garden where God created us and placed us. However, we

2. Haraway, *The Companion Species Manifesto*, 9.

claim that this garden is not some primeval plot of perfection that we seek to recreate, but it is in *this world* where God resides and holds all things together. Our ecclesiological visions must be both congruent with the descriptions we have offered of what it means to be bodyselves and at the same time spark imaginative and creative images of who we will become together as the body of Christ.

According to Genesis, God plants a garden and places humans in it. I have no idea what kind of gardener God was. We know that the garden was not perfect, maybe even a tad messy. The word "perfect" is not used to describe the garden or the humans that God created. Within the garden, Adam is joined by animals as companions and Eve as his partner. All created by God. Later on in the familiar story, God is taking an evening walk and asks Adam and Eve, "Where are you?" Either God can't find Adam and Eve because the garden is a mess or it's a rhetorical question. God asks us the same question: Where are you? Do we know? We are in God's creation and to reply with anything different than this is an inadequate response to the question. We are in God's creation because we are creatures. And creatures can be quite wild and messy.

Wildness and messiness abound in the garden described by Haraway. We look everywhere around us in this garden and can't distinguish what is natural from artificial, cultural from natural, plant from animal, human from nonhuman. I'm fairly sure that most of what I eat is a combination of genetically modified crops—probably corn and soybeans. The beef that I eat on rare occasion is probably from a cow that ate genetically modified feed. We are the created co-creators of a planet on which nothing escapes human technological intervention. The animals in this techno-garden are companions in my home, ones that I eat, and others, which are used for research. The characters that live in this garden are messy, hybrid, and complex.

I grew up learning that humans are the exception in our world, that we are not only different from but also superior to all the other creatures on this planet. In this worldview, humans are at the center of the universe, at least from their perspective. But modern science tells us otherwise. We are as much a part of the garden as any other creature, and furthermore, the fact that we recognize this creates a moral obligation for us to get along with the others.[3] Since the animals with which I am the closest are dogs, I find

---

3. Haraway writes: "The Great Divides of animal/human, nature/culture, organic/technical, and wild/domestic flatten into mundane differences—the kinds that have

it appropriate to reflect on their difference and yet similarity to me and to reflect on what I have learned about living with them as my companions.[4]

The worst thing I can do to them is to not recognize that they are dogs, and not furry children. To not respect their *dogness* is to disrespect that they are in relationship to me. Dogs are bred to provide human companionship. Humans are, however, not dog. And that distinction is critical. If I only treat dogs from my perspective and needs, I don't respect them. This lesson I have learned from my dogs also works in many other relationships. Learning to respect others is a prerequisite for loving others as fellow companions along the way. Compassion and companionship are two sides of the same coin of love.

We learn this respect by listening to and learning from one another's bodyselves. In some delightful reflections from the *New York Times*, Dana Jennings writes about his "becoming" dog with his dog. In a rather odd little entry, he explains how he "became dog" when he went through treatment for cancer: "But after surgery, you're reduced to a helpless animal state. I needed to be fed and watered. And, when you're walking the hospital, your I.V. pole is effectively a leash. Bijou and I have both wrestled with issues of incontinence—though I never peed on anyone's foot."[5] If we get to know our companion canine does that lead us to knowledge about who we are? I believe it does. Jennings develops compassion with his incontinent dog, Bijou, because he has experienced the same thing in his own bodyself.

Jennings believes he has learned more than just physical lessons with his dog. He has also learned spiritual lessons when he developed with Bijou what he calls his "inner dog." He writes:

> I also learned that cancer time and dog time aren't so different. We know that our dogs' lives are compressed into ten to fifteen years that their brilliant flames burn even more quickly than our own. Time is compressed, too, when you have cancer, and even after. You can't take ten years from now for granted or next year for that matter. During all of this, Bijou has been a kind of accidental canine Zen master. The more I watch her, the more I learn. And the more I learn, the more I understand my inner dog.[6]

---

consequences and demand respect and response—rather than rise to sublime and final ends," *When Species Meet*, 15.

4 Haraway states: "Because we have never been the philosopher's human, we are bodies in braided, ontic and antic relating," *When Species Meet*, 165.

5 Jennings, "My Life as a Dog," par. 6.

6 Ibid.

How do we as companion species come together? We learn from our dogs through our shared fleshly experiences, respecting our distinct otherness. The more we listen and watch each other, the more we love each other.

When I play with my two large dogs, I enter into a different zone with them. I must meet the dogs on their own terms—as human to dog, not as a human who constructs a vision of what "dog" must be. Consequently, only through the step-by-step playing and training between my dogs and me, does the understanding of who dog is and who human is happen. Our love for one another emerges when we play with one another, when we abandon our expectations of what should happen and simply let our joy for one another be. What if, just what if, we learned to be church learning to play with one another, when we abandon our expectations of what should happen and we simply rejoice in one another? Our words could become flesh through the practices and play we call church. What better way to do this than to celebrate the ways we live together.

HOSPITALITY

What is hospitality? It is the experience of offering and receiving grace that goes above and beyond; it exceeds all expectations. With this definition in mind, we can explore what this might mean for being church through Scripture, medicine, healthcare. What does Scripture say?:

> The alien who resides with you shall be to you as the citizen among you: you shall love the alien as yourself; for you were aliens in the land of Egypt: I am the Lord your God. (Lev 19:34)

> There is nothing better for mortals than to eat and drink, and find enjoyment in their toil. This also, I saw, is from the hand of God; for apart from him—who can eat or who can have enjoyment. For to the one who pleases him God gives wisdom and knowledge and joy; but to the sinner he gives the work of gathering and heaping, only to give to one who pleases God. This also is vanity and a chasing after wind. (Eccl 2:24–26)

Hospitality is an exchange of God's love between self and other and between God and the world. Joy and delight mark the hospitable exchange, creating new relationships.

One of the best descriptions of hospitality that I have come across is used in the context of medicine and healthcare. Sociologist Arthur Frank suggests that the relationship of host and guest, generosity and hospitality is a model for how we can get along with one another. He explains that to face an illness like cancer requires that the person will need to learn to be a body in new ways so that he or she can face unknown fears, confront pain, and mourn the loss of good health. Such relearning takes time, trust, and grace. He calls this medical generosity: "My book is about what I consider fundamental medicine: face-to-face encounters between people who are suffering bodily ills and other people who need both the skills to relieve this suffering and grace to welcome those who suffer. Medical generosity lacks in the latter quality—the grace to welcome those who suffer."[7]

Using language that has spiritual overtones, Frank describes the relationship of guest and host as generosity in action. This happens when we are most vulnerable, when we are sick and afraid of what might happen. What if not only our healthcare communities could model those values through their practices of generosity, but also our churches? Recovering the radical hospitality of the relationship between host and guest means that the host must also become the guest. Then hospitality is an experience of grace. Baptism and Eucharist can be those radical sacramental acts that challenge traditional exclusions of which bodies can belong in the body of Christ, and the sacraments open the body of God to all. Hospitality then is amazing grace.

A few years ago, I experienced such grace and hospitality that it changed my life. Gary, my husband, and I became friends with Arthur and Rosemary Peacocke from Oxford, England. Arthur had two PhDs—one in biochemistry and one in theology. I knew Arthur through the times we had met at religion and science dialogues and over the course of time we became friends. Several times the four of us met—whether in Sioux Falls or Oxford. Meals, long wonderful meals, were the times when we enjoyed each other's company and took time with each other. Even when we ate breakfast at their home, we did so with silver napkin rings and fresh flowers on the table. Some might consider this as proper British manners, but we experienced it as extravagant hospitality. When I wrote a book with Arthur, he delighted in serving fine Sherry—a habit that more American academics should cultivate. However, a few years ago, Arthur was diagnosed with cancer and it spread to his bones.

On one trip to Oxford, I had a poignant experience of spending time in a British hospice for a day or two where Arthur was receiving pain

---

7. Frank, *The Renewal of Generosity*, 1.

medication. The hospice was a round building, with magnificent glass windows and an inner courtyard filled with gardens. The trolley cart delivered sherry during happy hour, and patients with lung cancer were allowed to smoke in the beautiful gardens. The extravagant hospitality of life was given for those who were dying. In the last days while Arthur was dying, his doctor suggested that he write his final words. Arthur's last words in his book published posthumously were about experiencing the love of God. He wrote: "Over the years I have given much thought and spilt much ink on the nature of God and God's interaction with people. Not surprisingly the subtle nuances of my deliberations have fallen away before the absolute conviction that God is love and eternally so. This remains the foundation of my prayers and thoughts for 'underneath are the everlasting arms.'"[8]

Arthur's honesty about his dying freed me to share my grief and loss. Even in his final months and days, he was host to my grief. Amazing grace, indeed. So in his final days he wrote: "The irony is that one of the examples I took was the role of mutations in DNA which are the basic source of evolution, and so of the emergence of human beings—and also of cancer. This is a new challenge to the integrity of my past thinking. I am only enabled to meet this challenge by my root conviction that God is Love as revealed supremely in the life, death and resurrection of Jesus the Christ."[9] These are words of grace to me and others who can learn from Arthur that God's love for all of creation is indeed extravagant. When we find ourselves facing death, will we be ready for the extravagant love of God? Can I join with Arthur in knowing that "absolute conviction that God is love and eternally so?" Faith is letting go of our own stinginess and accepting the extravagant hospitality of God's love.

I also experienced radical hospitality when I served as interim campus pastor for a year at Augustana College at the Chapel of Reconciliation. A few years before, a group of students had written up their mission/welcome statement and we included it in the bulletin, posting it on the chapel door. Like Luther's Ninety-Five Theses, this welcome statement was written with grace, humor, and elegance:

> Litany: Augustana Congregation Welcome Statement
>
> L: Come to me,
> C: All who believe, all who wonder, and all who don't know what to think.

8. Peacocke and Clayton, *All That Is*, 192.
9 Ibid., 193.

All who are joyful, all who suffer, and all who are complacent;
All who are homosexual, or heterosexual, or bisexual, and all who simply don't know;
All who are male, all who are female, and all who are transgender.

L: Come to me,

C: All who are young, all who are old, and all who know no age;
All who are black, or white, or brown, or tan, or yellow, or purple, or blue, or red, and
All combination of hues.
All who give grades, all who receive grades, and all who wish there was a better way;
All who love, all who long to be loved, and all who do not know love.

L: Come to me,

C: All who are healthy and all who are unwell;
All who hurt and all who are hurting;
All who judge and all who are judged;
All who feel included and all who feel left out;

ALL: Come to Me, all. I will give you rest. Come as you are. You are Welcome![10]

I felt welcomed into this community and I hoped those who walked in the door of the chapel felt that way as well. As members of this congregation we tried to live up to our mission by trying to take this hospitality into the communities around us: through student-led worship at the prison, in Bible studies led in the dorms, by working at the local food pantry and kitchen, praying with and for those around the world. I believe that the way we live together as church already shows the shape of our church. The habits we practice create communities in which we live. If we live out of cynicism and stinginess our community looks like that. But if we live with grace and humor, humility and responsibility, we can hope to be both guest and host, as living sacraments of hospitality. Larry Rasmussen, a Lutheran ethicist, writes: "We can adapt and create governance and leadership practices, then, by answering questions like these: Do our practices welcome all to the table? Are the discriminating distinctions drawn between people in society considered of no account here, and who do we show that in the way we regulate our life together? Are the guests and in turn called to be the

---

10. Augustana College, "Augustana Welcomes All Faiths."

hosts?"[11] Several times during the year we asked ourselves: Did only certain people feel welcome in this Chapel of Reconciliation? Were we really embodying the mission of the congregation? Hospitality can be both difficult to practice and difficult to receive.

How can we turn churches into places of hospitality? For one thing, it helps if you can get into the front door. The doors of Augustana College's chapel exclude some people from entering on their own. Students who have a physical disability experience constant frustrations as they make their way across campus. Students who are in wheel chairs are not able to get into the door of the chapel. There is nothing to push by the door that automatically opens it. So, unless the students sit and wait for the door to be opened by someone else, they couldn't come into worship, or to pray, or even just to visit. I think of all those bodies that the church has not wanted to enter in its sanctuaries at some point in its history. In many institutional religious settings, people are excluded from becoming pastors, from leading worship, and from feeling welcome simply because of their sex, race, age, economic class, or sexual orientation. Creating a hospitable sanctuary must start from the very beginning so that all who enter are able to find their place, to make it their spiritual home. That's hard work, and takes practice. Compassion and hospitality are not concepts, but embodied actions. Compassion and hospitality might be the most important means by which we practice being who God intended us to be as the body of Christ.

EXCREMENTAL ECCLESIOLOGY

Two years ago at Augustana College, our illustrious campus pastor Paul Rohde preached a series of sermons with the title "flush" in them. The sermons were accompanied by the sounds of toilets flushing at appropriate or inappropriate moments, depending on who was running sound. Of course, Lutherans are known for having bodily references in their theology. I'm sure that some Lutheran theologians could hardly contain their joy when it was announced that "Luther's lavatory thrills experts. Martin Luther's supposedly great insight into justification by grace through faith occurred while he was on the toilet."[12] Dr. Treu, a Reformation scholar and archaeologist with the foundation that studies and maintains Luther's home, who helped to discover this great archeological find, comments: "there can be little doubt

11 Rasmussen, "Shaping Communities," 129.
12 BBC News, "Luther's Lavatory Thrills Experts," par 8.

the toilet was used by Luther, the radical theologian who argued for a more earthy Christianity, which regarded the entire human body—and not just the soul—as God's creation."[13] The flush is simply a modern day addition to excremental theology. Luther, trained in the theology and exegesis of the Hebrew Bible, argued with his opponents who claimed that God was too "clean" or "pure" to really engage in human flesh. For Luther, God was most fully God when God was most fully human.

A few years ago I heard a modern Hebrew Bible scholar give a lecture on body images in the Psalms. As one example, he used this wonderful hymn text by Isaac Watts:

> Blest is the man whose bowels move,
> And melt with pity to the poor;
> Whose soul, by sympathizing love,
> Feels what his fellow saints endure.
>
> His heart contrives for their relief
> More good than his own hands can do;
> He, in the time of gen'ral grief,
> Shall find the Lord has bowels too.
>
> His soul shall live secure on earth,
> With secret blessings on his head,
> When drought, and pestilence, and dearth
> Around him multiply their dead.
>
> Or if he languish on his couch,
> God will pronounce his sins forgiv'n;
> Will save him with a healing touch,
> Or take his willing soul to heav'n.[14]

I've had my student congregation sing this hymn. Individuals chuckle and look around to see if anyone feels as awkward about the text as they do. I remind them that the Victorians changed the language of Watts' text and made it "cleaner." Docetism was declared a heresy by the early church, but it's still alive and well in congregations. I wonder how people would react as they recite the words in the Nicene Creed from: when God came down and was incarnate and was made human. We, who are now techno-sapiens, hybrids of machine and flesh, must continue to reflect on what it means that God is incarnate in the world, in human flesh. To not continue such theological reflection on the meaning of the creeds for us today is to ignore

---

13 Ibid.
14 Watts, "Blest Is The Man Whose Bowels Move."

the ways that both the traditions and our flesh interact with each other to create new meaning. Would we, like those in the Victorian era, find offense with such language? I wonder why we never sing hymns, recite creeds, or listen to sermons that honestly reflect the realities of bodyselves in the twenty-first century? I'm not sure we are ready for God to be that human.

The Body of God is not just a metaphor. God's presence in the world is in our bodies. In the Lutheran tradition, we express this through the little Latin axiom: *finitum capax infiniti*. The finite, earthly stuff of creation bears or cradles the infinite. We confess this in the creedal reference to Chalcedon that Jesus is "like unto us in our humanity, like unto God in his divinity." Humanity and divinity are not polar opposites—rather they cradle each other. And our bodies, like the body of Christ, are not a static metaphor, but a living, moving, changing community of human persons. Our bodies are God's way of being God in the world. Precisely in our full humanity—in our sufferings, failures, and doubts, we are moved to be members of the body of Christ.

St. Paul mentions in his letter to the Corinthians that he hopes "the members may have the same care for one another. If one member suffers, all suffer together with it; if one member is honored, all rejoice together with it" (1 Cor 12:26). When we are moved by compassion, our bodies are physically and emotionally moved by the needs of our neighbor. Think of the times when we use the language, "I was moved by such and such." We feel compassion inside our bodies—we know deep down in our guts what it means to experience such love and empathy. For Luther, the church is a community of persons who must display compassion physically. The church is the living body of Christ—not some abstract doctrine, or a specific building, or even the institution. Church is not a "what" but a "who," that is, an assembly of people gathered for word and sacrament. When Christians worship, they share the words: the body of Christ given for you and the blood of Christ shed for you. To use Dietrich Bonhoeffer's famous dictum: "Jesus calls us not to a new religion, but to life."[15] We are called to be living sacraments for the world.

What is church? Throughout the Christian tradition, all kinds of metaphors were used to explain what that might mean: the family of God, the body of God, the priesthood of all believers, the communion of saints, an army, the bride of Christ, a flock, pilgrims on the way. The bodies of those in charge of the institutional church usually reflected the metaphors

---

15. Bonhoeffer, "Letters and Papers," 804.

that they used. Douglas John Hall, a contemporary North American theologian, reminds the established churches of the Northern Hemisphere that they should no longer cling to "absurd and outmoded visions of grandeur," and to let go of "triumphalistic dreams of majority status and influence in high places and ask themselves about the possibilities of witnessing to God's justice and love from the edges of empire."[16] He explains that when Jesus used metaphors to describe his "flock" or the reign of God, he used images of smallness: "salt, yeast, light—small things that can serve larger causes because they do not aim to become big themselves."[17] Whether it's the "small" images from Scripture, or metaphors from our own cultures that we use, we want to think about what church is and what it might be in new ways. We need everybody in order to do that.

Everyone from the Gospel writers to St. Paul seems to have trouble explaining what it means to be a part of the body of Christ, that God became flesh. So they use a kind of show-and-tell language: stories, poetry, humor, parables, dreams, letters, and dialogue. At one level, I agree with Hall that we need to let go of our triumphalistic ways of being church, but we also need to pay attention to the cultural voices around us and listen attentively to what they are saying about what it means to be human bodyselves. Poets, artists, bloggers, journalists, scientists help us with this.

An example for the visual arts is the famous 1987 photograph by Andres Serrano, entitled *Piss Christ*. A small, white crucifix is submerged in a murky, yellow-brownish fluid, alluding to the piss which supposedly surrounds the religious object. Philip L. Smith fiercely objected: "The Virginia Museum should not be in the business of promoting and subsidizing hatred and intolerance. Would they pay the KKK to do a work defaming blacks? Would they display a Jewish symbol under urine? Has Christianity become fair game in our society for any kind of blasphemy and slander?" Reverend Donald E. Wildmon complained: "I would never, ever have dreamed that I would live to see such demeaning disrespect and desecration of Christ. . . . Maybe, before the physical persecution of Christians begins, we will gain the courage to stand against such bigotry." And the late Sen. Jesse Helms harangued, "I do not know Mr. Andres Serrano, and I hope I never meet him. Because he is not an artist, he is a jerk. Let him be a jerk on his own time and with his own resources. Do not dishonor our Lord." In 1997 in Australia, two teens attacked the photo with a hammer and a gallery visitor

---

16 Hall, "Cross and Context," 8.
17 Ibid., 9.

who attempted to destroy the photo, threatened: "I'd just like to punch [Serrano] in the nose."[18]

But as *New York Times* art critic Michael Brenson states:

> ... Mr. Serrano struggles against inhibitions about the human body. His use of bodily fluids is not intended to arouse disgust but to challenge the notion of disgust where the human body is concerned.
>
> It is possible to see Mr. Serrano's use of bodily fluids as pure provocation. But you can also believe that Mr. Serrano views them as a form of purification. The fluids make us look at the images harder and consider basic religious doctrine about matter and spirit.
>
> They also raise the issue that was so crucial to the Byzantine Iconoclast Controversy of the eighth and ninth centuries: the relationship of an image to what it represents. The controversy was a bitter and profound debate about the nature of images and the problem of mistaking images for religious truths that could never be entirely incarnated.
>
> The photograph is clean and purified, the reliquary or shrine in which he clearly believes that the word about the body can be stored and spread.[19]

In the Christian tradition we have not only dared to call Jesus "Lord" but also "fully human." But if Jesus is fully human it follows that he of necessity had to urinate. *Piss Christ* is a visual, visceral reminder of Jesus own bodyself. It grieves me to think that for those who found the artwork offensive, I am guessing that they would find anything that alludes to the crass bodily nature of Jesus as gross and disgusting.

Equally offensive for many Christians is *Christa*, the female crucifix sculpted by Edwyna Sandys displayed in New York's St. John the Divine Cathedral (Episcopal) in 1984. One initial negative response, by Richard Dillon of Fordham University's Religion Department, was slightly muted: "As a piece of art, it has every right to claim our attention. But as a devotional object, it has a responsibility to tradition."[20] The then two Suffragan Bishops of New York responded very negatively with Bishop Walter D.

---

18. Image of *Piss Christ* in Sutton, "A Brief History"; Smith quote cited in ibid., par. 2; Wildman quote in ibid., par. 3; Sen. Helms quoted in ibid., par. 5; Australian attack discussed in Art Crimes, "Piss Christ," par. 2.

19. Brenson, "Review/Art; Andres Serrano," pars. 13–5, 18.

20. Dillon, cited in Churcher and Murphy, "Intelligencer," 13.

Dennis stating "[*Christa* is] symbolically reprehensible" and "theologically and historically indefensible." Bishop Dennis had no problem with "enhancing" symbols of Jesus by using differing skin colors or ethnicities, but he objected to *Christa* "totally changing the symbol." Bishop J. Stuart Wetmore complained: "It does not surprise me someone, somewhere would do such a sculpture either out of cynicism, smart-aleckness or a distorted devotion."[21]

Perhaps the most absurd response to *Christa* has been by conspiracy-seeking Roman Catholic Dennis L. Cuddy, who understands *Christa* as the invasion of paganism, Freemasonry, and the New Age into the Catholic Church.[22] Conservative Roman Catholic blogger Evelyn Birge Vitz was distressed that in using images such as *Christa* "modern secular culture has moved increasingly toward demands for 'justice' for women—and away from the roles of wifehood and motherhood . . . [thus embracing] androgyny . . . [and abandoning] gender identity as having any theological significance at all."[23] Perhaps one of the more illogical and extreme reactionary responses to Sandys' sculpture was that of conservative Roman Catholics Mary J. and Leon Podles, who essentially rant that Christians have become "intent on emasculating God," using an "androgynous God." They question:

> *Why is God the Father* a father and not a mother? Maleness is a symbol of transcendence because the fundamental male experience, that of fatherhood, of reproduction through ejaculation, is one of separation, while the fundamental female experience is one of prolonged and intimate union with the offspring through the long months of gestation and nursing. The male experience of the world is one of "either/or," "this, and not that," one of separation.[24]

Southern Baptist theologian Curtis Scott Drumm understands Christians to "have abandoned the arts to the non-believing world and . . . the theological fringe." Therefore current "'religious' art" [is] works such as Edwina Sandy's *Christa* . . . ."[25]

Almost twenty years later, the group "Renew: A Women's Ministry Network for United Methodists" objected to various actions by the United Methodist Church's Women's Division of the General Board of Global

---

21. Both bishops cited in Briggs, "Cathedral Removing Statue," pars. 5–6, 21.
22. Cuddy, "The Catholic Church."
23. Birge Vitz, "God and the Sexes," par. 14.
24. Podles and Podles, "The Emasculation of God," pars. 3 and 10, their emphasis.
25. Drumm, "Putting God in a Frame," 21–2.

Ministries, including the mention of *Christa* in a Methodist publication.[26] This statement The Confessing Movement considered as one of many examples of the Women's Division of "theological misdirection and narrow, partisan, leftist perspectives."[27] And just a couple of years ago, Baptist theologian J. Carl Laney, who believes in scriptural infallibility and inerrancy, confuses the historical understanding of Jesus with the theological and devotional appropriation of Jesus: "It is quite clear from Scripture that Jesus Christ was a male. The angel Gabriel announced that Mary would 'bear a son' (Luke 1:31). Luke recorded that Mary 'gave birth to her first-born son' (2:7). The idea of a female Christ is indefensible biblically and historically. In His incarnation, Jesus Christ, the second person of the Trinity, is clearly male."[28] In light of these reactions to *Christa*, is it no wonder that some people still find the image of a woman presiding at the Eucharist to be offensive?

But as seminary professor, artist, and art gallery director Deborah reflected in a sermon after seeing *Christa* in an art gallery:

> What did viewers see when they looked at this piece of art? Some saw ugliness, heresy and blasphemy. Some visitors to the exhibition called *Christa* an abomination, at once a challenge to the immutable truth that Jesus was a man and a pornographic invitation towards the further abuse of women. Others called it bad art, a cheap trick, its chunky surface masking an unwillingness to deal carefully with anatomy, its too-obvious reference to two thousand years of Christian art an unacceptable visual shorthand in service to a polemic point. Still others found in it great beauty, truth, and even comfort as they considered a vision of Christ that said that Jesus' self-giving was not about his gender, but rather his humanity. For these viewers, the *Christa*, along with the rest of the show, seemed to say that wherever women are being abused, there Christ is still being crucified. For those who recognized the truth of its proclamation, the *Christa*'s very ugliness was a kind of beauty, a revelation of divine compassion.[29]

I don't know of many congregations who would want either the photograph or the crucifix as a centerpiece for their sanctuary. The artwork and

---

26. Renew Network, "OUR BASIS FOR CONCERN," par. 8. under "IV. Questionable Theological Teaching and Social Justice Mission Concept."

27. Ibid., par. 9 under "Opening Statement."

28. Laney, "Is God a He or a She," par. 3.

29. Sokolove, "Come and See," par. 9.

statues in many congregations portray the kind of Christ that the members want to worship: clean, white, and male, with nice long hair. While this clean and tidy God might appear as one who is easy to worship, in fact, "his" appearance does not reflect the realities of our messy bodyselves. Maybe every church, for a period of time, should hang either *Christa* or "Piss Christ" at the front and center in the sanctuary to remind them what it really means to be part of the body of Christ. Otherwise our theology is not worth flushing.

IMPROVISATION

To be part of an improvisational ensemble, a community of players requires discipline and attentive listening. To learn how to improvise involves tending to our bodies' rhythms and movements. We learn them through practice with others. Improvisation is an event, a process within a group of people. Improvisation is learning to adapt. The ways we move along the way is who we become as an ensemble. Music helps our bodies remember, to be of "full accord" and share the "same mind." Anything that creates memories also creates rituals. Improvisation starts with listening, working with what you already have. And if church is to be an ensemble, we start with our traditions and adapt them for the world in which we currently live. Improvisation requires learning, practicing, listening and it's much more than doing "your own thing." In fact, improvisation can only happen within communities. We need not only care what traditions we hand down, but also how they are handed on to others. Music and the other arts provide a model for learning how to do this.

Music and the arts are universal expressions of human experience, allowing for multiple cultural variations. Music goes beyond words and creates resonance with life experiences. Just think of the various ways that monastic communities through the practice of lectio divina use the Psalms. Pottery and the visual arts also sustain different ways of knowing and remembering within our bodies. The arts can radically change the environment of our lives. When we learn about another culture, we learn about their music, visual arts, foods, and other habits. When we learn another language we often do so by learning about their customs. I remember learning hymns and other songs and poetry when I learned Latin. I can still remember a few of the Latin words to "Rudolph the Red-Nose Reindeer." Our bodies learn to speak the language through the music—the rhythms and scales. And these are often different across cultures. Instead of merely being told about the differences between cultures, our bodies can learn them by participating in them. We almost seem wired for music.[30] All of creation participates in the music of life. I think of the example where Mozart supposedly composed a piece based on a tune that his deceased starling sang. Music is idiomatic and conveys the idiosyncratic customs of creatures and cultures.

In Scripture there is a lot of singing, dancing, and eating. When I ask people what it means to belong to a certain religion, I find that people list their favorite hymns, or Bible passages that they have memorized, or liturgical rituals that define special moments in life. Some of the controversies in churches have been over seemingly insignificant changes in the way we practice our beliefs: how we commune or where the baptismal font is placed. But if these rituals are as deeply embodied and ritualized as I think, then I understand why change can be so traumatic. I think of college students who are often longing for the familiar amidst the chaos of their daily lives. When I suggested changing the Lord's Prayer to the newer translation, I met with stalwart opposition. "No." That's going too far, I was told. In the chaos of their lives, they needed something to hold on to, something familiar. Our bodies know our traditions—through how to kneel or when to receive communion, or what smells are in the sanctuary. Each tradition carries different postures that convey their theological positions. Do you sign yourself with the cross? Do you kneel or stand at communion?

These bodily practices both unite and divide us. I've had several conversations that remind me how difficult it is to be in the body of Christ—for we are often a body that is fragmented and torn apart. Many of us knew all too well how painful it has been to be a part of the Evangelical Lutheran Church in American as we discussed and voted in a new statement about sexuality. For the first time, gay, lesbian, transsexual, transgender people in committed partnerships would be ordained. Some people celebrated, others left. Communion becomes another dividing point within the church. Families have been split in half over who can commune or be baptized in which denomination. And yet these differences are more like strict divisions—they fragment and hurt the body of Christ. To make it worse, many of these divisions are manifestations of certain parts of the body wanting more power than others. We create a kind of us/them theology that divides the body of Christ and shatters the love of God.

30. For an entertaining introduction to this issues see Sacks, *Musicophilia*.

We call each other names: conservative, liberal, heretic, and orthodox. What can we do with these divisions? In St. Paul's epistle to Corinth, he addresses a church that is much like the contemporary scenes I just described where differences turn to divisions that tear apart the body of Christ:

> For just as the body is one and has many members, and all the members of the body, though many, are one body, so it is with Christ. For in the one Spirit we were all baptized into one body—Jews or Greeks, slaves or free—and we were all made to drink of one Spirit. Indeed, the body does not consist of one member but of many. On the contrary, the members of the body that seem to be weaker are indispensable, and those members of the body that we think less honorable we clothe with greater honor, and our less respectable members are treated with greater respect; whereas our more respectable members do not need this. But God has so arranged the body, giving the greater honor to the inferior member, that there may be no dissension within the body, but the members may have the same care for one another. If one member suffers, all suffer together with it; if one member is honored, all rejoice together with it. (1 Cor 12:12–14, 22–26)

Corinth was a major metropolitan center of trade, tourism, and religious pilgrimage. And the community was marked by great diversity: Jew/Greek, slave/free. And these differences would often turn into hurtful divisions. This is the context in which Paul writes the chapter about love. Amidst the painful and hurtful divisions we create, Paul calls upon us to love one another. It is important to note that Paul's words are to a specific congregation with specific issues—and so these famous words about love are not about some generic, feel-good, happy-clappy love—but instead are a counter-cultural proclamation and address specific people who are hurting. God's love for us and our love for one another must address the particular situations we find ourselves in. That's the tough part about this text and about being church. These are words of tough love for hurting people. Healing the Body of God is not easy. So, how can we turn division into a unity of diverse people who all are part of the body of Christ?

I don't know. But I have one idea. I was telling my husband about struggling to write a sermon on the passage from 1 Corinthians 12 and he said, "You should look back at the Rule of St. Benedict."[31] I knew exactly what he meant. We have spent time in the Benedictine communities and have found that they are very, very diverse and yet they learn to live in

---

31. St. Benedict, "The Rule of St. Bendict"; also many print editions.

community with one another as one body of Christ. The first word in the rule of St. Benedict is: *listen*. This simple and yet profound insight from the Rule of Benedict offers a beginning point for interpreting Paul's words about love to the community of Corinth and to us. We will need to learn to "listen with the ear of our heart," and not with pre-conceived stereotypes. Being a part of the body of Christ, is realizing that our part is not the whole part . . . that we are just that—a part. "God loves us, and hates you" is sin. But love leads to wholeness and reconciliation is a faithful response. And practicing the act of love is that—a practice. Church is sharing practices of faith with each other over time. Participating in the body of Christ means creating intentionally complex relationships practiced over time. The radical message of grace, that the body of Christ is broken for all of creation, must be shared in the sanctuaries, but also, and even more importantly, out in service to and with the world. The Christian community is formed by the way it is composed, practiced, and performed. Let's hope that our compositions have multiple tonal centers, many different players, and celebrate the diverse "themes" of the Christian heritage.

ANAMNESIS

Anamnesis happens in both religion and medicine. It is the practice of recalling events that shape and empower the present. Physicians practice anamnesis when they listen to and help a patient to tell their story. In the Christian tradition, liturgical leaders recall the saving acts of God and then during the Eucharistic liturgy create ways for the congregants to enter into and participate in the paschal mystery of faith. In both examples, recall and memory are physical processes of the individual and of the community. We make the past come to life when remembering through rituals of the present. When we remember and share our life stories with one another, we encounter the sacred.

The way I have learned a great deal about anamnesis and about being part of church is from a group of women that I met with every Monday afternoon at three o'clock. We gathered in a large office in the Chapel of Reconciliation on campus. The sun often warmed the space and we began with coffee and tea, and usually told a few personal anecdotes from the preceding week. This writing group was for anyone who had cancer or who either knew someone or who had a family member or friend that had cancer. We were a motley crew bound together by an illness, but also by friendships that formed over the course of our writing together for several months. Our group had a physician, an ethicist, staff and faculty from the college, a student, and a retired teacher. Dr. Mary Helen Harris, an emergency medicine physician and professor at the Sanford School of Medicine at the University of South Dakota, led the group in our writing exercises each week. Mary Helen has attended workshops on teaching writing for those in the professions, particularly healthcare.

So, adapting what she learned from this setting, Mary Helen gave us our writing prompt for the day. One word. We then spent a few minutes, around twenty or so, writing. At the end of our sessions, we gathered the writings that we wanted to share and we evaluated them to see how the process and product of the writing has (hopefully!) led to insights about spiritual transformation and about our relationships. Our goal was to compare the similarities and differences of each other's journeys in order to gain more insight about the experience of cancer. What has happened, however, was unpredictable. Some began the journey through cancer years ago, others had barely started. Some were in the middle of treatment; others had experienced the loss of a loved one. We talk about new innovations in the treatment of cancer, what foods most likely make one vomit after chemotherapy, and remember ways that healing can occur.

Our stories were more like scripts, written and rewritten for every new context and time we met. Some of the themes remain constant. We talk about our bodies, the parts that had cancer, and the hair that has fallen out and grown back in quirky new ways. Each week we learned more about cancer, our spiritual journey, and our selves. The stories emerged, coming together in bits and pieces, weaving past and future into our present moment. Anamnesis. Being and becoming church.

PILGRIMS ALONG THE WAY

Central to the life of the church is the ecology of how it functions as a human community. By "ecology," we mean how its parts fit together, how they work. The internal ecology of the church is located within a larger ecology—that of the world around it. The church is a subsystem within the larger ecosystem. One way to imagine this relation of the internal and external ecology is to think of the church as a community on a journey, making its way through the landscape in which it has been placed; we might also say a pilgrim community, a community on the way, expressed classically in the term *communio viatorum*. We always seek to understand how the parts of our community relate to each other and recognize what ways of relating are most desirable—this is our internal "ecology." We are also always trying to comprehend how our community should relate to the terrain of our journey—this is the exterior ecology. The two work together, inseparable within a large, dynamic living reality. Whether we look inward or outward, ours is ecology of immigrants tracking a changing landscape. The challenge is to understand how the church can maintain itself as a community that is engaged in this tracking of the terrain over which it moves.

The images of *journey* and being *on the move* are deeply etched on the church's consciousness. God's call to Abraham and Sarah was to be on their way, and their journey away from the settled, "golden" city of Ur was credited to them as righteousness (Rom 4:22). To be the "people of God" was synonymous in the Old Testament with breaking camp and moving on in response to God—into Egypt, out of Egypt in the exodus, forty years in the wilderness. It was only when the conquest of Canaan appeared on their horizon that Israelites developed an image of an earthly "homeland."

Those early centuries of Israel's existence mirrored the 40,000 years of human pre-history—prior to the emergence of agriculture 10,000 years ago—when being human meant always being *on the way*. That was the way of life, and survival depended on it—moving seasonally to follow the game that provided our food; migrating in the face of the frequent changes in climate—south when the ice sheets encroached, north when they receded. And, of course, before we were Europeans, Middle Easterners, or Asians, we were Africans. Our pre-history was a very long trek that lasted for many generations.

The followers of Jesus were called "people of the way" in the earliest years; that moniker is remembered in the traditional image of "the community on the way," the "community of pilgrims" (*communio viatorum*). Today, being *on the way* is as fundamental to human identity and Christian identity as it has ever been. The millions of people who were compelled to leave their homelands in the twentieth century and in the first decade of the present century know this very well. Millions more of us in the USA are children and grandchildren of migration—whether from other lands or other regions in the US. We miss the point when we label migrants "transients" or when we judge them negatively as "lawbreakers."

All too easily, the church may forget that being on the way is fundamental to being church—but in these days we are being reminded, because

God is calling us, like Abraham and Sarah, to leave the settled homes of our Ur and to move on; God's history always moves on. As Christians, we believe that the journey is God's. God's Spirit undergirds us and the terrain we traverse. We learn more about God as we travel—surprised at every turn by God's unexpected moves. For the ELCA, the journey is both literal and metaphoric. Geography is part of it—out of the center city and some efforts to go back in; out of the rural regions; into the suburbs; out of the northeast and upper Midwest, into the Sunbelt and the west; frequently away from the working classes and into the more affluent classes; globalization brings the entire world into our lives, often with jarring consequences; the contrast between rich and poor demands attention. A new interfaith reality compels us to rearrange our ideas of what constitutes true religion. Ethnicity and demographics are also part of our journey: from Scandinavian and German to African American, Latino, Asian, and Native American Indian. Descendants of the original Lutheran immigrants join with people who have migrated from other denominations to the ELCA.

Mores change on the journey as well—lesbian, gay, and transsexual along with straight; single parent and blended families adding to traditional nuclear families; divorce as well as life-long unions. Culture is central—rock music, rap, hip-hop, and jazz along with Bach and Handel. Science and technology totally condition our lives, including the practice of medicine. Our medicine enables life at its beginning and extends it until life's end—*in vitro* fertilization and embryo reduction, premature babies, preserving eggs and sperm for future fertilization. We cure illness through transplants, sometimes with tissue from other species, and stem cell research. Life is extended through all manner of means, a transhuman mentality that puts off death for as long as possible. Electronic communication shapes our personal interactions: Internet and iPhone, Facebook and Twitter; Kindle alongside printed books and newspapers. We frequently overlook that every one of these migrations in electronic communication is affecting our life in the ELCA, even if we do not understand them very well or ignore them.

Being on the way means that we are always immigrants tracking this changing landscape; it means that we must know that terrain, and know it very well. We must develop our powers of imagination as we figure out where God is in this journey and how we can live as the people of God in this terrain—that's the challenge. All of this takes place in the dynamic and power of God's Spirit. The journey is God's, and so is the terrain. The Spirit undergirds the knowledge and imagination we need for this journey. We believe that the Word of God in Jesus Christ reveals the meaning of our journey. We trust that God will give us the insight and courage we need. In the present situation, our pilgrim faith is being tested as never before.

We are wanderers, pilgrims on the way. We need to have a willingness to let go. We move from one location in the past for somewhere new in the future. We are on the threshold and crossing into new and strange places. We are on the threshold of who we are becoming as church. Hopefully, we move from confusion and uncertainty to maturity of openness. What does it mean to be a people "on the move"? When we are the body of Christ, we are called to bear witness to each other's suffering and to listen. We must listen with our whole person, not just our minds, but also our whole selves, fully attentive to the words, to the facial expressions, to the tone of the voice of the other. The body of Christ makes a way out of no way when people are healed; captives are set free, and dark yesterdays are transformed into bright tomorrows. Belonging to the body of Christ is being called to action. Making a way out of no way is not about theory, but about practice, making a way out of no way is not just an ideal, but a real transformation. Transformation happens with other people by the Spirit of God's power alive in us: "let us remember that there is a creative force in this universe, working to pull down the gigantic mountains of evil, a power that is able to make a way out of no way and transform dark yesterdays into bright tomorrows. Let us realize the arc of the moral universe is long but it bends toward justice."[32]

Church is about life along the way, an incarnational pilgrimage. Being and becoming the church needs to be about a radical experiment of living that way—about that community, about providing freedom from the constraints of our crazy lives that limit our being open to others and to God. We must discover God and church along the way—and we may find it in magic moments sharing food and drink, in compassionate embraces with those who suffer, in the companion animals who share our lives, and through the hard work and adventuresome play of daily life. We aren't church already; we become church along the way. Church is both particular within the bodies of Christ that we are and cosmically as we partake in the larger body of God. Creation is the community in which we are church.

---

32. King, "Where Do We Go From Here?," last par. The final phrase "moral arc of the universe..." originated with the nineteenth century Unitarian minister, abolitionist, and social reformer Theodore Parker in his sermon "Of Justice and the Conscience," 84–85.

There is no other "place," no other "church." We are God's bodyself: created, loved, and redeemed.

Afterword

WE BEGAN BY SAYING that this book would offer no comprehensive, conceptually spelled out view of the body, and we kept that promise. Rather we have offered a series of *takes* on the body—from different angles, caught up in a variety of movements, simple and complex, straightforward and yet at the same time defying comprehension. These takes need follow no particular order—you can dip into the book at any chapter.

You may wish we had provided more about the body, but we hope you will agree that what is here is authentic, pertinent, fascinating, and produces endless chains of questions. We invite you, the reader, to pick up from here, offering your own takes on your body, all the bodies you know, all that you think about.

We leave the reader with a series of pithy statements; all together, they provide our final take:

Not everything is body, but our bodies ultimately lead us into everything that can be thought and experienced. Even things that we can never experience are brought to mind by our bodies.

Our brains are as much our body as our arms and legs and hearts and livers. In our thinking and feeling, our body is the active agent. When we think about our body, it is our body thinking about itself. Trying to understand our body is an exercise in self-understanding.

Our bodies are nature, in their evolutionary history and in their present outreach. Our bodies compel us to reflect on how we think of nature. And what we think about nature touches on everything we think about: ourselves, other people, the world around us, God, life, love, death, life after death.

Our bodies contain our life-stories. We have a history and we have been many places. When we tell our story, it is our body telling its story.

Afterword

We've shared a few snapshots of our body-stories here. It makes no sense to think of our life-stories as separate or abstracted from our bodies.

Our faith and our theology include our bodies in ways we had never thought of before. Even our beliefs about Jesus Christ relate in amazing ways to what we believe about bodies.

Our bodies are selves—bodyselves. God created us this way.

S.B
P.H
A.M.P

Suggestions for Further Reading

CHAPTER 1. A NEW PARADIGM: BODY-SELF

Bartlett, Jennifer, et al. *Beauty Is a Verb: The New Poetry of Disability.* El Paso, TX: Cinco Puntos, 2011.

Sanford, Matthew. *Waking: A Memoir of Trauma and Transcendence.* Emmaus, PA: Rodale, 2006.

CHAPTER 4. DISCOVERING OUR CULTURE'S SCRIPT

Noe, Alva. *Out of Our Heads: Why You Are Not Your Brain, and Other Lessons from the Biology of Consciousness.* New York: Hill & Wang, 2010.

Turkle, Sherry. *Alone Together: Why We Expect More from Technology and Less from Each Other.* New York: Basic, 2011.

Winterson, Jeanette. *Written on the Body.* New York: Vintage International, 1994.

CHAPTER 6. WHERE MEDICINE AND CHRISTIANITY COLLIDE

Frank, Arthur. *The Wounded Healer: Body, Illness, and Ethics.* Chicago: University of Chicago Press, 1995.

Montross, Christine. *Body of Work: Meditations on Morality from the Human Anatomy Lab.* New York: Penguin, 2007.

Weiner, Jonathan. *His Brother's Keeper: A Story from the Edge of Medicine.* New York: HarperCollins, 2004.

CHAPTER 7. A SCIENTIFIC TAKE ON OUR BODYSELVES

Bennett-Woods, Deb. *Nanotechnology: Ethics and Society.* Boca Raton, FL: CRC, 2008.

Boysen, Earl, and Nancy D. Muir. *Nanotechnology for Dummies: A Fun and Easy Way to Explore the Science of Matter's Smallest Particles.* Hoboken, NJ: Wiley, 2011.

Suggestions for Further Reading

Fagan, Brian. *Cro-Magnon: How the Ice Age Gave Birth to the First Modern Humans*. New York: Bloomsbury, 2010.
Pääbo, Svante. *Neanderthal Man: In Search of Lost Genomes*. New York: Basic, 2014.
Powers, Richard. *Generosity: An Enhancement: A Novel*. New York: Picador 2000.
Shubin, Neil. *Your Inner Fish: A Journey into the 3.5-Billion-Year History of the Human Body*. New York: Pantheon, 2008.
Skloot, Rebecca. *The Immortal Life of Henrietta Lacks*. New York: Crown, 2010.
Waal, Frans de. *Good Natured: The Origins of Right and Wrong in Humans and Other Animals*. Cambridge: Harvard University Press, 1996.
Wenz, John. "The Other Neanderthal," *The Atlantic*. No pages. Online: www.theatlantic.com/technology/archive/2014/08/the-other-neanderthal/375916/.
Wilson, E. O. *On Human Nature*. Cambridge: Harvard University Press, 1978.

CHAPTER 8. THE HUMAN JOURNEY

Hefner, Philip. "Biocultural Evolution and the Created Co-Creator." In *Science and Theology: The New Consonance*, edited by Ted Peters, 174–88. Boulder, CO: Westview, 1998.
———. "Going As Far As We Can Go: The Jesus Proposal For Stretching Genes and Cultures." *Zygon: Journal of Religion and Science* 34 (1999) 485–500.
Menzel, Peter, and Faith D'Aluisio. *Robosapiens: Evolution of a New Species*. Cambridge: MIT Press, 2000.

CHAPTER 9. NATURE, MYSTERY, AND GOD

Collingwood, C. G. *The Idea of Nature*. Oxford: Oxford University Press, 1945.
Corrington, Robert. *Nature and Spirit: An Essay in Ecstatic Naturalism*. New York: Fordham University Press, 1992.
Peacocke, Arthur. *All That Is: A Naturalistic Faith for the Twenty-first Century*. Edited by Philip Clayton. Minneapolis: Fortress, 2007.

CHAPTER 10. LUTHER ON THE BODY: INCARNATION, TECHNO-SELF, AND FAITH

Rolvaag, Ole. *Giants in the Earth: A Saga on the Prairie*. New York: Harper Perennial Modern Classics, 1999.
Solberg, Mary M. *Compelling Knowledge: A Feminist Proposal for an Epistemology of the Cross*. Albany, NY: State University of New York Press, 1997.
Sponheim, Paul R. *The Pulse of Creation*. Minneapolis: Augsburg Fortress, 2000.

Suggestions for Further Reading

CHAPTER 11. THE BODY OF CHRIST

Bolz-Weber, Nadia. *Pastrix: The Cranky, Beautiful Faith of a Sinner & Saint.* New York: Jericho, 2014.

Clayton, Philip. *Transforming Christian Theology: For Church and Society.* Minneapolis: Fortress, 2009.

Bibliography

Aarnoudse-Moens, Cornelieke Sandrine Hanan. "Meta-Analysis of Neurobehavioral Outcomes in Very Preterm and/or Very Low Birth Weight Children." *Pediatrics* 124 (2009) 717–28.
The African Queen. Directed by John Huston [1951]. DVD. Hollywood, CA: Paramount, 2010.
Alexander, Richard. *The Biology of Moral Systems*. Hawthorne, NY: de Gruyter. 1987.
Alfonsi, Sharyn, and Ursula Fahy. "In Search of Love: Teens Lured into Sex Trade," Sept. 22, 2010, ABCNews.com. Online: http://a.abcnews.com/US/portland-emerges-hub-child-sex-trafficking/story?id=11690544&singlePage=true.
Alvarez, Lizzette. "Spirit Intact, Soldier Reclaims His Life." *New York Times*, July 2, 2010. Online: http://www.nytimes.com/2010/07/04/nyregion/04soldier.html?pagewanted=all&_r=0.
American Society of Plastic Surgeons. "2012 Plastic Surgery Statistics Report." ASPS National Clearinghouse of Plastic Surgery Procedural Statistics April 22, 2013. Online: http://www.plasticsurgery.org/Documents/news-resources/statistics/2012-Plastic-Surgery-Statistics/full-plastic-surgery-statistics-report.pdf.
Ammons, A. R. "Poetics." In *Collected Poems: 1951–1971*, 199. New York: Norton, 1972.
Art Crimes. "Piss Christ." Online: http://www.artcrimes.net/piss-christ#fn2.
The Associated Press. "8 facts about 'Octomom' Nadya Suleman." January 24, 2014. Online: http://www.usatoday.com/story/news/nation/2014/01/24/8-facts-octomom/4816235/.
Augustana College. "Augustana College Welcomes All Faiths." Online: http://www.augie.edu/augustana-welcomes-all-faiths.
Aziz, Khalid. "NRP Current Issues Seminar: Case-Based Discussion on Neonatal Ethics," October 30, 2013, American Academy of Pediatrics. Online: http://www2.aap.org/nrp/docs/Fri%20209%200100%20Collura%20Aziz%20Ringer%20NRP%20Ethics%20Session.pdf.
Babette's Feast [Karen Blixen's *Babettes gæstebud*]. Directed by Gabriel Axel [1987]. Santa Monica, CA: MGM Home Entertainment, 2001.
Bakker, Robert T. *Raptor Red*. New York: Bantam, 1995.
Bartlett, Jennifer, et al. *Beauty Is a Verb: The New Poetry of Disability*. El Paso, TX: Cinco Puntos, 2011.
Bazell, Robert. *Her-2: The Making of Herceptin, a Revolutionary Treatment for Breast Cancer*. New York: Random House, 1998.

Bibliography

BBC News. "Luther's Lavatory Thrills Experts." Online: http://news.bbc.co.uk/2/hi/3944549.stm.

Beck, Stacy, et al. "The Worldwide Incidence of Preterm Birth: A Systematic Review of Maternal Mortality and Morbidity." *Bulletin of the World Health Organization* 88 (2010) 31–38.

Behrman, Richard E., and Adrienne Stith Butler, eds. *Preterm Birth: Causes, Consequences, and Prevention*. Committee on Understanding Premature Birth and Assuring Healthy Outcomes. Washington, DC: National Academies Press, 2007.

Bell, Catherine M., and Reza Aslan. *Ritual: Perspectives and Dimensions*. Rev. ed. New York: Oxford University Press, 2009.

Benedict of Nursia, Saint. *The Rule of St. Benedict*. Online: http://www.ccel.org/ccel/benedict/rule.i.html; http://christdesert.org/Saint_Benedict/Study_the_Holy_Rule_of_St__Benedict/index.html.

Beniger, James R. "Piss Christ," COMM 544: Arts and the New Media. Online: https://www.usc.edu/schools/annenberg/asc/projects/comm544/library/images/502.html.

Bennett-Woods, Deb. *Nanotechnology: Ethics and Society*. Boca Raton, FL: CRC, 2008.

Birge Vitz, Evelyn. "God and the Sexes" September 1, 1995. Online: http://www.crisismagazine.com/1995/god-and-the-sexes-2.

Birkerts, Sven. "Emerson's 'The Poet'—A Circling." *Poetry 100* (April 2012) 69.

Blencowe, Hannah, et al. "National, Regional, and Worldwide Estimates of Preterm Birth Rates in the Year 2010 with Time Trends since 1990 for Selected Countries: A Systematic Analysis and Implications." *The Lancet* 379 (2012) 2162–72.

Bonhoeffer, Dietrich. *Ethics. Dietrich Bonhoeffer Works*, Vol. 6. Edited by Clifford J. Green and translated by Ilse Tödt. Minneapolis: Fortress, 2008.

———. "Letters and Papers from Prison, July 16, 1944." In *The Bonhoeffer Reader*, edited by Clifford J. Green and Michael P. DeJonge, 749–818. Minneapolis: Fortress, 2013.

Bolz-Weber, Nadia. *Pastrix: The Cranky, Beautiful Faith of a Sinner & Saint*. New York: Jericho, 2014.

Boysen, Earl, and Nancy Muir. *Nanotechnology for Dummies*. 2nd. ed. Hoboken, NJ: Wiley, 2011.

Brenson, Michael. "Review/Art; Andres Serrano: Provocation and Spirituality." *New York Times*, December 8, 1989. Online: http://www.nytimes.com/1989/12/08/arts/review-art-andres-serrano-provocation-and-spirituality.html?pagewanted=2&src=pm.

Brick, M. "And Next to the Bearded Lady, Premature Babies." *New York Times*, June 12, 2005. Online: http://www.nytimes.com/2005/06/12/nyregion/12coney.html.

Briggs, Kenneth A. "Cathedral Removing Statue of Crucified Woman." *New York Times*, April 28, 1984. Online: http://www.nytimes.com/1984/04/28/nyregion/cathedral-removing-statue-of-crucified-woman.html.

Burnett, Leo. "The Marlboro Story: How One of America's Most Popular Filter Cigarettes Got that Way." *The New Yorker* 34, November 15, 1958, 41–43. Online: Legacy Tobacco Document Library, University of California San Francisco Library, http://legacy.library.ucsf.edu/tid/zea48d00/pdf;jsessionid=658EDFF1CF5F86EC8C46ABCBD8958C01.tobacco04.

———. Interviewed by Kathleen Schalch. "Present at the Creation: The Marlboro Man." October 21, 2002. Online: http://www.npr.org/templates/story/story.php?storyId=1152015. Audio online: http://www.npr.org/player/v2/mediaPlayer.html?action=1&t=1&islist=false&id=1152015&m=152015.

Bibliography

Cacioppo, John T., and William Patrick. *Loneliness: Human Nature and the Need for Social Connection.* New York: Norton, 2008.

Callison, Jill. "Embracing the Church: Transgender Minister to be Received as ELCA Pastor." Online: http://revrohrer.blogspot.com/2010/07/in-news-argus-leader.html.

Camponesi, Silvia. "Oscar Pistorius, Enhancement and Post Humans." *Journal of Medical Ethics* 34 (2008) 639.

CanWest News Service. "Miracle Child." February 11, 2006. Online: http://www.canada.com/topics/bodyandhealth/story.html?id=db8f33ab-33e9-429f-bedc-b6ca80f61bdc.

Cash, Johnny. "Folsum Prison Blues." *Johnny Cash at Folsom Prison*, track 1. Compact disc recording. The American Milestones Series. New York: Columbia/Legacy, 1999.

Chemnitz, Martin. *De Duabus Naturis in Christo* . . . . Np: n.d.

Chessman, Harriet Scott. *Lydia Cassatt Reading the Morning Paper.* New York: Seven Stories Press, 2001.

Child, Lee. "Lee Child Bibliography." N.d. Online: http://leechild.com/images/uploads/Lee-Child-Bibliography.pdf.

Churcher, Sharon, and Mary Murphy. "Intelligencer." *New York Magazine* 17.18, April 30, 1984, 13.

Clark, Andy. "Curing Cognitive Hiccups: A Defense of the Extended Mind." *The Journal of Philosophy* 104.4 (2007) 163–92. Online : http://www.journalofphilosophy.org/articles/104/104-4.htm#.

Clayton, Philip. *Transforming Christian Theology: For Church and Society.* Minneapolis: Fortress, 2009.

Collingwood, Robin George. *The Idea of Nature.* 1945. Reprint. Eastford, CT: Martino Fine Books, 2014.

Connolly, Katie. "Six Ads That Changed the Way You Think." BBC News, January 3, 2011. Online: http://www.bbc.co.uk/news/world-us-canada-11963364.

Coneyislandhistory.org. "Roslyn Tromer: Incubator Baby." Online: http://www.coneyislandhistory.org/voices/index.php/Voices/SetDetail/set_id/9.

Corrington, Robert. *Nature and Spirit: An Essay in Ecstatic Naturalism.* New York: Fordham University Press, 1992.

Costleloe, Kate L., et al. "Short Term Outcomes after Extreme Preterm Birth in England: Comfson of Two Birth Cohorts in 1995 and 2006 (the EPICure studies)." *British Medical Journal* 345 (December 2012) e7976. Online: http://www.bmj.com/content/345/bmj.e7976.long.

Council of Chalcedon. "Chalcedonian Decree." In *Christology of the Later Fathers*, edited by Edward Hardy in collaboration with Cyril Richardson, 371–74. Philadelphia: Westminster, 1954.

Crowley, Paul. "Tomorrow's Theologians." *America* 204.3, February 7, 2011, 9.

Crichton, Michael. *Prey: A Novel.* New York: HarperCollins, 2003.

Cuddy, Dennis L. "The Catholic Church, Freemasonry, and the New Age." Online: http://www.dailycatholic.org/issue/2002Apr/apr16btf.htm

Curtis, Bryan. "The Curious Case of Lee Child: Before Tom Cruise Could Become Jack Reacher, Jim Grant Had to Become Lee Child," *Grantland*, December 20, 2012. Online. http://grantland.com/features/lee-child-jim-grant-jack-reacher/.

Dargis, Manohla. "Millions of Friends, but Not Very Popular." *New York Times*, September 24, 2010. Online: http://www.nytimes.com/2010/09/24/movies/ 24nyffsocial.html?_r=0, September 23.

Bibliography

Davidson, Lela. "Ultrasound Parties New Frontier Pregnancy Oversharing." January 2, 2013, The Today Show Parenting. Online: http://www.today.com/parents/ultrasound-parties-new-frontier-pregnancy-oversharing-1C7753058.

Davincisurgery.com. "Features." Online: http://davincisurgery.com/da-vinci-surgery/da-vinci-surgical-system/features.php.

De Grey, Aubrey. Curriculum Vitae [2012]. 18 pages. Online: http://www.sens.org/sites/srf.org/files/AdG-CV.doc.

Departures. Directed by Yojiro Takita. Henley, UK: Arrow Films, 2008.

Dillon, Richard, SSL., cited in Sharon Churcher and Mary Murphy, "Intelligencer," *New York Magazine* 17.18, April 30, 1984, 13. Online: https://books.google.com/books?id=f-UCAAAAMBAJ&pg=PA13&lpg=PA13&dq=edwina+sandys+christa&source=bl&ots=yF-NzPoKBv&sig=j7d5cIiK2FnvoTFYz Mf5M_TqTtQ&hl=en&sa=X&ei= oTSnVIXEPM62oQT-iYLABQ&ved=oCBoQ6A EwADgU#v=onepage&q= edwina%20sandys%20christa&f=false.

Drumm, Curtis Scott. "Putting God in a Frame: The Art of Rene Magritte as Religious Encounter." Ola Farmer Lenaz Lecture, December 13, 2001, New Orleans Baptist Theological Seminary. Online: http://www.baptistcenter.net/papers/Drumm_Putting_God_in_a_Frame.pdf.

Eliot, T. S. "The Hippopotomus." In *The Complete Poems and Plays*, 50. New York: Harcourt, Brace, 1950.

Evangelical Lutheran Church in America and Evangelical Lutheran Church in Canada. "Evening Prayer." *ELW*, 309–19.

———. "Night Prayer. *ELW*, 320–7.

———. "Prayer at the Close of the Day." *ELW*, 154–63.

———. "Responsive Prayer." *ELW*, 161–3.

Fagan, Brian. *Cro-Magnon: How the Ice Age Gave Birth to the First Modern Humans.* New York: Bloomsbury, 2010.

Farjeon, Eleanor. "Morning Has Broken." Hymn 556 in *Evangelical Lutheran Worship* by Evangelical Lutheran Church in America and Evangelical Lutheran Church in Canada. Minneapolis: Augsburg Fortress, 2006.

Fjermedal, Grant. *The Tomorrow Makers: A Brave New World of Living-Brain Machines.* New York: MacMillan, 1986.

Frank, Arthur W. *The Renewal of Generosity: Illness, Medicine, and How to Live.* Chicago: University of Chicago Press, 2004.

———. *The Wounded Healer: Body, Illness, and Ethics.* Chicago: University of Chicago Press, 1995.

Fukuyama, Francis. *Our Posthuman Future: Consequences of the Biotechnology Revolution.* New York: Farrar, Straus and Giroux, 2002.

Goldberg, Michelle. "The Super Bowl of Sex Trafficking." *Newsweek*, January 30, 2011. Online: http://www.newsweek.com/super-bowl-sex-trafficking-66681.

Gornick, Vivian. *The Situation and the Story: The Art of Personal Narrative.* New York: Farrar, Straus and Giroux. 2001.

Graham, Jorie. "At Luca Signorelli's Resurrection of the Body." In *Erosion*, 76–7. Princeton: Princeton University Press, 1983.

———. "At Luca Signorelli's Resurrection of the Body." Online: http://www.smith.edu/poetrycenter/poets/atlucas.html.

Hall, John Douglas. "Cross and Context: How My Mind Has Changed." *The Christian Century* 127.18, September 7, 2010, 34–40.

Bibliography

Hamilton, W. D. "Evolution of Altruistic Behavior." *American Naturalist* 97 (1963) 354–6. Online: http://greatergood.berkeley.edu/images/uploads/Hamilton-EvolutionAltruisticBehavior.pdf.

Haraway, Donna Jeanne. *The Companion Species Manifesto: Dogs, People, and Significant Otherness*. Chicago: Prickly Paradigm, 2003.

———. *Modest_Witness@Second_Millennium. FemaleMan_Meets_OncoMouse: Feminism and Technoscience*. New York: Routledge, 1997.

———. *When Species Meet*. Posthumanities 3. Minneapolis: University of Minnesota Press, 2008.

Hayes, Zachary. *A Window to the Divine: A Study of Christian Creation Theology*. St. Bonaventure, NY: Franciscan Institute, 1997.

Hefner, Philip. "Biocultural Evolution and the Created Co-Creator." In *Science and Theology: The New Consonance*, edited by Ted Peters, 174–88. Boulder, CO: Westview, 1998.

———. "Going As Far As We Can Go: The Jesus Proposal for Stretching Genes and Cultures." *Zygon* 34 (1999) 485–500.

———. "The Knitter." Unpublished poem, 2012.

———. "Living in Paradox." Unpublished poem, 2014.

———. *Technology and Human Becoming*. Facet Books. Minneapolis: Fortress, 2003.

———. "Teilhard's Spiritual Vision of the Mystical Milieu." In *The Legacy of Pierre Teilhard de Chardin*, edited by James Salmon, 79–94. Mahwah, NJ: Paulist, 2012.

———. "To the Knitter." Unpublished poem, 2012.

———. "When the Angel Kneads Harshly." Revision of Rainer Maria Rilke, "The Man Beholding," translated by Robert Bly. January 18, 2014. Online: http://philnevahefner.wordpress.com/2014/01/18/when-the-angel-kneads-harshly/.

Hendel, Kurt K. "*Finitum Capax Infiniti*: Luther's Radical Incarnational Perspective." *Currents in Theology and Mission* 35.6 (2008) 420–33.

Hopkins, Gerard Manley. "God's Grandeur." In *The Poems of Gerard Manley Hopkins*, 4th ed., edited by W. H. Gardner and N. H. MacKenzie, 66. New York: Oxford University Press 1967.

———. "God's Grandeur." Online http://www.poetryfoundation.org/poem/173660.

Howson, Christopher, Mary Kinney, and Joy Lawn, eds. *Born Too Soon: The Global Action Report on Preterm Birth*. Geneva: World Health Organization, 2012. Online: http://www.who.int/pmnch/media/news/2012/201204_borntoosoon-report.pdf.

Huxley, Julian. *Evolution: The Modern Synthesis*. 1942. Reprint. Cambridge: MIT Press, 2010.

———. "Transhumanism." *In New Bottles for New Wine*, 13–7. London: Chatto & Windus, 1957. Online: http://www.transhumanism.org/index.php/WTA/more/huxley.

Irons, William. "How Did Morality Evolve?" *Zygon* 26 (1991) 49–89.

Ishiguro, Kazuo. *Never Let Me Go*. New York: Knopf, 2005.

Javier, Annie. "Jumping to Premature Conclusions." *Virtual Mentor: American Medical Association Journal of Ethics* 10 (2008) 659–64. Online: http://virtualmentor.ama-assn.org/2008/10/pfor2-0810.html.

Janvier, Annie, et al. "The Experience of Families with Children with Trisomy 13 and 18 in Social Networks." *Pediatrics* 130.2 (2012) 293–8. Online: http://pediatrics.aappublications.org/content/130/2/293.full.pdf+html.

Bibliography

Jennings, Dana. "My Life as a Dog," *New York Times*, September 15, 2009. Online: http://well.blogs.nytimes.com/2009/09/15/finding-my-inner-dog-through-cancer/?_php=true&_type=blogs&_r=0.

Keene, Ann T. "Pilates, Joseph Hubertus." American National Biography. Oxford: American Council of Learned Societies, Oxford University Press, 2008, online update October 2008. Online. http://www.anb.org/articles/19/19-00980.html.

Kierkegaard, Søren. *Concluding Unscientific Postscript*. Translated by David Swenson and Walter Lowrie. Princeton: Princeton University Press, for the American-Scandinavian Foundation, 1941.

———. *Philosophical Fragments or A Fragment of Philosophy*. Translated by David Swenson. Princeton: Princeton University Press, for the American-Scandinavian Foundation, 1936.

King, Martin Luther Jr. Speech to the Southern Christian Leadership Council, Atlanta, Georgia. August 16, 1967. Online: http://mlk-kpp01.stanford.edu/index.php/encyclopedia/documentsentry/where_do_we_go_from_here_delivered_at_the_11th_annual_sclc_convention.

King, Mary-Claire. "Introduction." In *Her-2: The Making of Herceptin, a Revolutionary Treatment for Breast Cancer* by Robert Bazell, xi–xiv. New York: Random House, 1998. Online: http://www.mayoclinic.org/breast-cancer/herceptintherapy.html.

Kingsolver, Barbara, with Steven L. Hopp and Camille Kingsolver. *Animal, Vegetable, Miracle: A Year of Food Life*. First Harper Perennial ed. New York: HarperCollins, 2007.

Kismet Project. "Overview." Online: http://www.ai.mit.edu/projects/sociable/overview.html.

Knight, Christopher. *The God of Nature: Incarnation and Contemporary Science*. Theology and the Sciences. Minneapolis: Fortress, 2007.

Kuner, Susan, and Carol Orsborn, Linda Quigley, Karen Stroup. *Speak the Language of Healing: Living with Breast Cancer without Going to War*. Berkeley, CA: Conari, 1999.

Lady Gaga [Stefani Germanotta], singer; Lady Gaga [Stefani Germanotta] and Jeppe Laursen, lyricists; Fernando Garibay and Paul Blair, producers. "Born this Way." On *Born This Way*, Audio CD, track 2. Santa Monica, CA: Streamline, Interscope, Kon Live, 2010.

Lady Gaga [Stefani Germanotta], performer, Nick Knight director. *Born this Way*. Music video. Online: http://www.mtv.com/videos/lady-gaga/742058/born-this-way.jhtml, 2011.

Lantos, John. *The Lazarus Case: Life-and-Death Issues in Neonatal Intensive Care*. Baltimore: Johns Hopkins University Press, 2001.

Levertov, Denise. "An Interim." *Poems 1968–1972*. New York: New Directions, 1987.

Lambert, Mary, Ben Haggerty [Macklemore], and Ryan Lewis, performers; Mary Lambert, Ben Haggerty [Macklemore], and Ryan Lewis, lyricists; Ryan Lewis, producer; "Same Love." On *The Heist*, audio CD, track 5. Seattle: Macklemore & Ryan Lewis, 2012.

Laney, J. Carl. "Is God a He Or a She?" November, 11, 2013. Online: http://www.westernseminary.edu/transformedblog/2013/11/19/is-god-a-he-or-a-she/.

Lelwica, Michelle Mary. *The Religion of Thinness: Satisfying the Spiritual Hungers behind Women's Obsession with Food and Weight*. Carlsbad, CA: Gürze, 2009.

Leo the Great, "The Tome of Leo." In *Christology of the Later Fathers*, edited by Edward Hardy in collaboration with Cyril Richardson, 359–70. Philadelphia: Westminster, 1954.

Bibliography

Luther, Martin. *Martin Luther on the Bondage of the Will. A New Translation of De Servo Arbitrio (1525) Martin Luther's Reply to Erasmus of Rotterdam*. Translated by J. I. Packer and O. R. Johnston. Westwood, NJ: Revell, 1957.

———. "To the Christian Nobility of the German Nation." Translated by Charles M. Jacobs; revised by James Atkinson. In *Three Treatises*, 1–112. Minneapolis: Fortress, 1970.

Madonna [Madonna Louise Ciccone], performer; Peter Brown and Robert Rans, lyricists; Nile Rodgers, Madonna [Madonna Louise Ciccone], and Stephen Bray, producers, "Material Girl," on Madonna, *Like a Virgin*, audio CD, track 1. Burbank, CA: Sire, 1984.

Marchese, John. "A Rough Ride." *New York Times*, September 13, 1992. Online: http://www.nytimes.com/1992/09/13/style/a-rough-ride.html?pagewanted=all.

Martin, Joyce A., et al. "Births: Final Data for 2012." *National Vital Statistics Reports* 62.9, 2013. Division of Vital Statistics, National Center for Health Statistics: Hyattsville, MD, 2013.

Meadow, William, and John Lantos. "Moral Reflections on Neonatal Intensive Care." *Pediatrics* 123.2 (2009) 595–7.

Menzel, Peter, and Faith D'Aluisio. *Robosapiens: Evolution of a New Species*. Cambridge: MIT Press, 2000.

Miles, Margaret. "'The Rope Breaks When It Is Tightest': Luther on the Body, Consciousness, and the Word." *HTR* 77:3–4 (1984) 239–58.

Montross, Christine. *Body of Work: Meditations on Mortality from the Human Anatomy Lab*. New York: Penguin, 2007.

Moravec, Hans. *Mind Children: The Future of Robot and Human Intelligence*. Cambridge: Harvard University Press, 1988.

Murphy, Nancy. "From Neurons to Politics—Without a Soul." In *Neuroethics: An Introduction with Readings*, edited by Martha J. Farah, 357–64. Cambridge: MIT Press, 2010.

Nanji, Ayaz. Associated Press, "World's Smallest Baby Goes Home." February 8, 2005. Online: http://www.cbsnews.com/news/worlds-smallest-baby-goes-home/.

NBCNews.com. "Actor Who Played in Ads Dies from Smoking-Related Disease." January 27, 2014. Online: usnews.nbcnews.com/_news/2014/01/27/22459778-actor-who-played-marlboro-man-in-ads-dies-from-smoking-related-disease?lite.

Niebuhr, H. Richard. *Christ and Culture*. New York: Harper. 1951.

Noe, Alva. *Out of Our Heads: Why You Are Not Your Brain, and Other Lessons from the Biology of Consciousness*. New York: Hill and Wang, 2009.

Now I Lay Me Down to Sleep. "Family Testimonials." Online: https://www.nowilaymedowntosleep.org/families/family-testimonials/.

Nuffield Council on Bioethics. *Critical Care Decisions in Fetal and Neonatal Medicine: Ethical Issues*. London: Nuffield Council on Bioethics, 2006. Online: http://nuffieldbioethics.org/project/neonatal-medicine/

Owen, D. R. G. *Body and Soul, a Study on the Christian View of Man*. Philadelphia: Westminster, 1956.

Pääbo, Svante. *Neanderthal Man: In Search of Lost Genomes*. New York: Basic, 2014.

Parikh, Rahul K., MD. "In Preemies, Better Care Also Means Hard Choice." *New York Times*, August 13, 2012. Online: http://www.nytimes.com/2012/08/14/health/views/better-care-for-premature-babies-also-means-harder-choices.html?_r=1&.

Bibliography

Parker, J. Ryan. "Gaga Does God's Work." *Pop Theology: Where Religion Meets Culture*, February 17, 2011. Online: http://www.patheos.com/blogs/poptheology/2011/02/born-this-way/.

Parker, Theodore. "Of Justice and the Conscience." *Ten Sermons of Religion*, 66–102. Boston: Crosby, Nichols, 1853. Online: https://archive.org/details/tensermonsofreliooinpark.

Parker's Bistro. "Parker's Vibe." Online: http://www.parkersbistro.net/ParkersonMain/Parkers_Vibe.html [accessed about September 2010, page now changed].

Patient Safety Canada. "Circumstances of Baby's Death Revealed during Healthcare Collaboration with Family," 2012. Online: http://www.patientsafetyinstitute.ca/English/news/PatientSafetyNews/Pages/Circumstances-of-baby%E2%80%99s-death-revealed-during-healthcare-collaboration-with-family.aspx.

———. "The Patient Narrative—Barb Farlow." October 29, 2013. Online: http://www.youtube.com/watch?v=XliZGuhHqx4.

Paul, Annie Murphy. *Origins: How the Nine Months before Birth Shape the Rest of Our Lives*. New York: Free Press, 2010.

Peacocke, A. R., and Philip Clayton. *All That Is: A Naturalistic Faith for the Twenty-first Century: A Theological Proposal with Responses from Leading Thinkers in the Religion-Science Dialogue*. Theology and the Sciences. Minneapolis: Fortress, 2007.

Pearce, Matt. "At Least Four Marlboro Men Have Died of Smoking-Related Diseases." *Los Angeles Times*, January 27, 2014. Online: http://www.latimes.com/nation/nationnow/la-na-nn-marlboro-men-20140127-story.html.

Pederson, Ann Milliken. *The Geography of God's Incarnation: Landscapes and Narratives of Faith*. Eugene, OR: Cascade, 2013.

———. "Ongoing Reformation." Online: https://byronandjack.wordpress.com/2013/04/24/ongoing-reformation/. In response to Dannika Nash, "'I Said I Don't Know'—and Other Answers to Hard Questions, 'An Open Letter to the Church from My Generation.'" Online: http://dannikanash.com/2013/04.

Perlman, Jeffrey M., et al., "Special Report—Neonatal Resuscitation: 2010 American Heart Association Guidelines for Cardiopulmonary Resuscitation and Emergency Cardiovascular Care." *Pediatrics* 126 (2010) e1319–44. Online: http://pediatrics.aappublications.org/content/126/5/e1319.full.html.

Phillips, J. B. *Your God Is Too Small*. 1945. Touchstone edition. Reprint. New York: Simon & Schuster, 2004.

Picoult, Jodi. *My Sister's Keeper: A Novel*. A Washington Square Press trade paperback edition. New York: Washington Square, 2009.

Pilates Foundation. "The History of Pilates." Online: http://www.pilatesfoundation.com/pilates/the-history-of-pilates/

P!nk [Alica Beth Moore], Max Martin, and Shellback. "Raise the Glass." Track 16 on *P!nk. Greatest Hits—so Far!!!*, CD audio recording, track 17. [United States]: LaFace Records, 2010.

P!nk [Alica Beth Moore]. "Raise Your Glass," official video. Directed by Dave Meyers. Online: https://www.youtube.com/watch?v=XjVNlG5cZyQ.

Podles, Mary, and Leon J. "The Emasculation of God." 2010. Online: http://www.podles.org/The-Emasculation-of-God.htm.

Pollan, Michael. *The Botany of Desire: A Plant's Eye View of the World*. 2001. Paperback. New York: Random House, 2002.

Powers, Richard. *Generosity: An Enhancement*. New York: Farrar, Straus and Giroux, 2009.

Bibliography

Prasad, R. "A Little Miracle Called Madeline." *The Hindu*. August 26, 2004. Online: http://www.thehindu.com/seta/2004/08/26/stories/2004082600411400.htm.

Quint Boenker Preemie Survival Foundation. "Preemie Survival." http://preemiesurvival.org/info/index.html.

Rahikh, R. "In Preemies, Better Care Also Means Hard Choice." *New York Times*, August 13, 2012. Online: http://www.nytimes.com/2012/08/14/health/views/better-care-for-premature-babies-also-means-harder-choices.html.

Renew Network, "OUR BASIS FOR CONCERN: A Brief Recounting of Questionable Actions on the part of the Women's Division of the General Board of Global Ministries," A White Paper Prepared by the RENEW Network, December 2001. Online: http://www.ucmpage.org/articles/umw_white_paper.html#reImagining.

Ricoeur, Paul. *The Rule of Metaphor: Multi-Disciplinary Studies in the Creation of Meaning in Language*. Translated by Robert Czerny with Kathleen McLaughlin and John Costello SJ. London: Routledge and Kegan Paul, 1978.

Rolvaag, Ole. *Giants in the Earth: A Saga on the Prairie*. New York: Harper Perennial Modern Classics, 1999.

Rosenfeld, Alfred, photos by Lennart Nillson. "Drama of Life Before Birth." *Life* 58.17, April 30, 1965, 54–71.

Sainte-Justine University Hospital. "Annie Javier." January 1, 2014. Online: http://recherche.chusj.org/en/Chercheurs/Bio?id=f8deb1fb-9bb5-4bed-b8be-a2d323731ac0.

Sakmari, Elvira, and Grant Stinchfield. "Pimps and Prostitutes Expected with Super Bowl XLV." January 3, 2011. Online: http://www.nbcdfw.com/news/local/Pimps-and-Prostitutes-Expected-with-Super-Bowl-XLV-110948159.html.

Sandford, Matthew. *Waking: A Memoir of Trauma and Transcendence*. Emmaus, PA: Rodale, 2006.

Santa Fe Institute. "About." Online: http://www.santafe.edu/about/.

———. "What Is Complex Systems Research?" Online: http://www.santafe.edu/about/faq/.

Schleiermacher, Friedrich. *The Christian Faith*. Translated by Hugh R. Mackintosh and J. S. Stewart. Edinburgh: T. & T. Clark, 1999.

Schmid, Heinrich Christo. Translated by Charles A. Hay, and Henry Eyster Jacobs. *The Doctrinal Theology of the Evangelical Lutheran Church*. 2nd rev. ed. Philadelphia: Lutheran Publication Society, 1889.

SENS Research Foundation. "Executive Team." Online: http://www.sens.org/about/leadership/executive-team.

Shanken, Andrew M. "Better Living: Toward a Cultural History of a Business Slogan." *Enterprise and Society* 7 (2006) 485–519.

Shubin, Neil. *Your Inner Fish: A Journey into the 3.5-Billion-Year History of the Human Body*. New York: Pantheon, 2008.

Siedell, Daniel A. "Haystacks and Shadow." Online: http://www.patheos.com/blogs/cultivare/2012/11/haystacks-shadows.

Sittler, Joseph. "Education as Furniture and Propellant." *The Christian Century*, February 3–10, 1988, 102–4. Online: http://josephsittler.org/articles/education.html.

Skloot, Rebecca. *The Immortal Life of Henrietta Lacks*. New York: Crown, 2010.

The Social Network. Directed by David Fincher. Culver City, CA: Sony Pictures Home Entertainment, 2011.

Bibliography

Sokolove, Deborah. "Come and See." A sermon preached January 16, 2005, at Seekers Church, Washington, D.C. Online: http://www.seekerschurch.org/worship/sermons/958-deborah-sokolove-come-*and-see*.

Solberg, Mary M. *Compelling Knowledge: A Feminist Proposal for an Epistemology of the Cross*. Albany, NY: State University of New York Press, 1997.

Sophie's Choice. Directed by Alan Pakula [1983]. DVD. Santa Monica, CA: Live Entertainment, 1999.

Sponheim, Paul R. *The Pulse of Creation*. Minneapolis: Augsburg Fortress, 2000.

Stout, Hilary. "Toddlers' Favorite Toy: The iPhone." *New York Times*, October 17, 2010. Online: http://www.nytimes.com/2010/10/17/fashion/17TODDLERS.html?pagewanted=all.

Strawson, Galen. *Selves: An Essay in Revisionary Metaphysics*. Paperback. Oxford: Clarendon, 2011.

Streiner, David L. "Attitudes of Parents and Health Care Professionals toward Active Treatment of Extremely Premature Infants." *Pediatrics* 108.1 (2001) 152–57. Abstract available online: http://pediatrics.aappublications.org/content/108/1/152.abstract.

Sutera, Judith, OSB, ed. *Work of God: Benedictine Prayer*. Collegeville, MN: Liturgical, 1997.

Sutton, Benjamin. "A Brief History of Piss Christ," December 25, 2013. *Bloun ArtInfo*. Online: http://blogs.artinfo.com/artintheair/2013/12/25/a-brief-history-of-piss-christ/.

Teilhard de Chardin, Pierre. *The Divine Milieu*. Harper Torchbooks. New York: Harper & Row, 1965.

———. "Mass on the World." In *Hymn of the Universe*, 9–33. Translated by Gerald Vann, OP. New York : Harper & Row, 1965.

———. "My Universe." In *Science and Christ*, 37–85. Translated by Rene Hague. New York: Harper & Row 1968.

Teilhard de Chardin, Pierre, et al. *The Phenomenon of Man*. New York: Harper & Row, 1961. Harper Torch Books. Online: https://archive.org/details/ThePhenomenonOfMan.

Temple, William. *Nature, Man and God; Being the Gifford Lectures Delivered in the University of Glasgow in the Academical Years 1932–1933 and 1933–1934*. London: Macmillan, 1935. Online: http://www.giffordlectures.org/Browse.asp?PubID=TPNMAG&Volume=0&Issue=0&ArticleID=26.

Tillich, Paul. "You Are Accepted." In *The Shaking of the Foundations*, 153–63. 1948. Reprint. Eugene, OR: Cascade, 2012.

———. *Systematic Theology*. Vol. 3. Chicago: University of Chicago Press, 1963.

Turkle, Sherry. *Alone Together: Why We Expect More from Technology and Less from Each Other*. New York: Basic, 2011.

Urban Dictionary. "Selfie." Online: http://www.urbandictionary.com/define.php?term=Selfie, definition 1, written 2009.

Waal, Frans de. *Good Natured: The Origins of Right and Wrong in Humans and Other Animals*. Cambridge: Harvard University Press 1997.

———, ed. *Tree of Origin: What Primate Behavior Can Tell Us about Human Social Evolution*. Cambridge: Harvard University Press 2002.

Watts, Isaac. "Blest Is The Man Whose Bowels Move." Online: http://www.hymnary.org/hymn/PHW/Ps.96.

Weiner, Jonathan. *His Brother's Keeper: A Story from the Edge of Medicine*. New York: HarperCollins, 2004.

Bibliography

Wenz, John. "The Other Neanderthal." *The Atlantic*. Online: www.theatlantic.com/technology/archive/2014/08/the-other-neanderthal/375916/.

Westendorff, Owen. "You Satisfy the Hungry Heart." *Evangelical Lutheran Worship*, hymn 484. The Evangelical Lutheran Church in America and the Evangelical Lutheran Church in Canada. Minneapolis: Augsburg Fortress, 2006.

Wikipedia: The Free Encyclopedia. "Nadya Suleman." Online: http://en.wikipedia.org/w/index.php?title=Special:Book&bookcmd=download&collection_id=ecbf8f45e83330914aafa87d6e1ef090769bad33&writer=rdf2latex&return_to=Nadya+Suleman http://en.wikipedia.org/wiki/Nadya_Suleman.

Wilson, Edward O. *Sociobiology: The New Synthesis*. 1975. Twenty-fifth anniversary ed. Cambridge: Belknap, 2000.

———. *Naturalist*. Washington, DC: Island Press [for Shearwater Books], 1994.

———. *On Human Nature*. Cambridge: Harvard University Press, 1978.

Winterson, Jeanette. *Written on the Body*. New York: Vintage International, 1994.

World Health Organization. "Global Health Expenditure Database." Online: http://apps.who.int/nha/database/Select/Indicators/en.

Wrangham, Richard. "The Evolution of Social Structure." In *Primate Societies*, edited by Barbara B. Smuts et al., 282–96. Chicago: University of Chicago Press, 1987.

Wrangham, Richard W., and Dale Peterson. *Demonic Males: Apes and the Origins of Human Violence*. Boston: Houghton Mifflin, 1996.

Yellow-Bird, Pemina. "Wild Indians: The Story of Canton Insane Asylum." Online: http://www.power2u.org/downloads/NativePerspectivesPeminaYellowBird.pdf.

Zahorsky, John. "Baby Incubators: A Study of the Care of Premature Infants in Incubator Hospitals Erected for Show Purposes. Part 1." *St. Louis Courier of Medicine* 31 (1904) 345–58. Online: https://archive.org/stream/stlouiscourierof3119unse#page/n364/mode/1up.

www.ingramcontent.com/pod-product-compliance
Lightning Source LLC
Chambersburg PA
CBHW052214240426
43670CB00037B/603